THE PERFECT RELATIONSHIP

SWAMI MUKTANANDA

The Guru
and
the Disciple

Translated by

Swami Chidvilasananda

PUBLISHED BY SYDA FOUNDATION

Published by SYDA Foundation
P.O. Box 600, South Fallsburg, New York 12779

Printed in the United States of America
Third printing, 1991

Cover design and art by Shane Conroy.

ISBN: 0-914602-53-5   LCCN: 80-54457

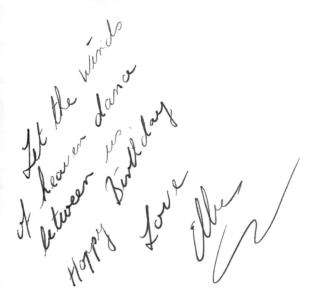

Let the winds
of heaven dance
between you.
Happy Birthday
Love

*I dedicate this book to the lotus feet of my supreme
father, Sadguru Bhagawan Nityananda, to whom I
owe my existence.*

CONTENTS

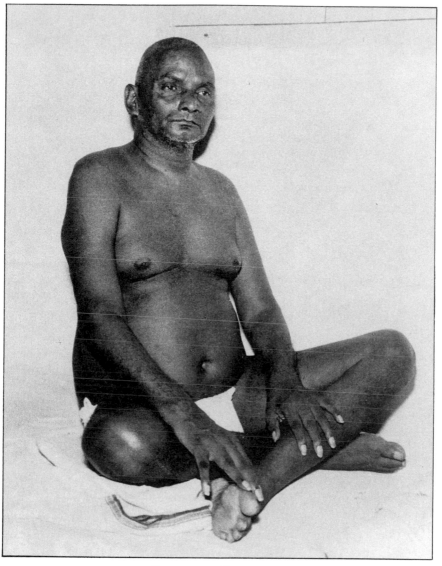

BHAGAWAN NITYANANDA

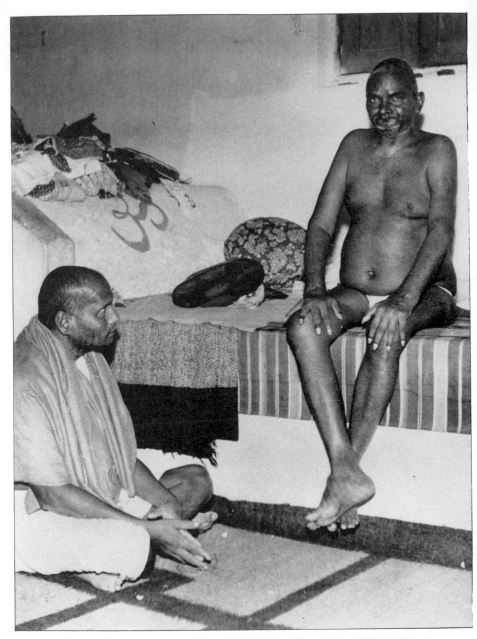

SWAMI MUKTANANDA WITH HIS GURU,   BHAGAWAN NITYANANDA

INTRODUCTION

Swami Muktananda speaks about the importance of chanting and mantra, of proper diet and a disciplined life. He speaks about meditation as a natural function of the mind: how every act of rapt attention is, in its way, a remembering of God. He has explained the nature of Kundalini, the coiled energy released by the spiritual process called *shaktipat*, which flows upward into a lotus-whiteness at the top of the head. He has told scriptural stories about Shiva, Shakti, and Krishna, drawing on the startling variety of an ancient tradition rich with gods and sages. Yet he never tires of repeating the simplest truth: "God dwells within you as you." God is not only the deity of a religious tradition, nor is he only a transcendent reality, a formless force. He is also the speechless interior of your own mind; he is consciousness; he is you in all your humanness, even all your faults and mistakes. Every avenue of Swami Muktananda's thought, every poem he sings and story he tells, brings us back to this simple knowledge which it is the mind's perverse tendency to forget and remember, over and over again.

Hearing Swami Muktananda speak about these and other matters, I have often felt that he was not speaking alone, for he was supported at all times by a memory, so strong it was almost visible, of his own Guru, Swami Nityananda. Twenty years after his Guru's death, Swami Muktananda existed in Nityananda's presence and never spoke except as his disciple. It occurred to me that this was the actual "secret" of Siddha Yoga and its essential wisdom, communicated not as an idea, but in the form of this daily, often subtle example.

Siddha Yoga is an ancient path, as old as human nature itself. It actually forms the basis of every tradition and, as Swami Muktananda eloquently explains, it is not a path that has much to do with techniques. Siddha Yoga comes to us from Siddhas, perfect beings, beings who are so completely rooted in their own Selfhood, in their inner God, that they see that God everywhere and can transmit their own experience to other people. Siddha Yoga is based on that act of communication. It is a yoga of relationship, founded on the knowledge, so obvious that we forget it all the time, that a human being lives most passionately and completely in the experience of love. Plato described a human being as an egg that was cut into halves long ago; now he runs everywhere looking to be whole again. We live in countless fleeting relationships, always seeking, finding, and losing again. As children and adults, we learn through these relationships. We learn by taking into ourselves our loved ones' thoughts and voices, absorbing our loved ones' very presence along with their knowledge.

After leaving home as a boy, Swami Muktananda traveled all over India. He studied Sanskrit and read the scriptures. He took the vows of a monk at the ashram of the great Siddharuda Swami. But his seeking led him further. Like the man in Plato's image, he longed to become whole again and sought the company of great beings wherever they resided: in ashrams, in forests, in cities, even on garbage heaps. He felt that God's "secret" was not contained in any Sanskrit formula, ancient ritual, or technique of meditation, that severe austerities and physical deprivation would not reveal it. He felt that the "secret" resided with great beings, with saints; they were themselves the "secret,"and he could learn what they were by loving them and sitting at their feet. After almost twenty-five years, he met Nityananda, who became his Guru. In a flash of self-understanding, he knew that he had found his other half, that now he was whole again. His true *sadhana* could begin because its goal was now definite and clear. He had discovered it in the fusing intensity of *shaktipat*—the transmission of Nityananda's spiritual energy—and also in the demanding, profoundly loving presence of his Guru.

All of Swami Muktananda's teaching amounts to this: If you want to become whole again, if you want to fulfill the quest that has occupied all your conscious loving life, seek a great being, a Siddha, with whom it is possible to have a perfect relationship. Fill your mind with his presence, become his disciple, until you have so absorbed his fearlessness and his love for God that you become what he is.

This is a book about that relationship. It is a book about the Guru, but it is equally a book about the disciple and about the spiritual journey itself. Swami Muktananda explains over and over again that only the Guru can point the way on this subtlest of all paths. "A person who walks in darkness does not know light. How can he look for light when he has never seen it?" Swami Muktananda asks in these pages. "If he tries to discover a path by himself, he will simply go around in circles, walking for a long time but never reaching his goal. . . Therefore, it is absolutely certain that you need a wise guide. . . The Guru has found everything you are seeking; that which you want has become the Guru's wealth. The difference between you and the Guru is that you are the seed and the Guru is the full-grown tree; you are the beginning, and he is the end. Inherently, the only difference between you is that one step."

This is the secret of the Guru-disciple relationship. The Guru *is* the disciple, but perfected, complete. When he forms a relationship with the Guru, the disciple is in fact forming a relationship with his own best self.

Swami Muktananda tells a story about a seeker who went to a Guru and asked him for instruction in the Truth. The Guru was a very simple, straightforward person, and when the seeker told him what he had come for, the Guru said, "Everything is Consciousness, and thou art That. That is the Truth."

"Is that all?" the seeker asked. "Can't you say anything more?"

"That is all I have to teach," the Guru said. "If you want something else, you'll have to go to another Guru."

The seeker left and eventually found his way to another Guru, who had a large ashram and many disciples. The seeker came to him and said, "I want to know the Truth. Please instruct me."

With a glance, the Guru understood what kind of seeker he was. "Have you been to see anyone else?" he asked.

The seeker named the other Guru. "All right," the Guru said, "I will give you instruction. But first you will have to serve me for twelve years." The Guru called his manager and asked him, "Have we any work for this seeker?"

The manager replied, "Every job in the ashram is filled except for one. We need someone to pick up cow dung in the cowshed."

"Will you do that job?" the Guru asked. The seeker agreed to do it, and so for the next twelve years he lived in the Guru's ashram, picking up cow dung in the cowshed. At the end of twelve years, he went to the Guru and said, "Twelve years are over. Please instruct me."

"Very good," said the Guru. "Here is my teaching: Everything is Consciousness, and thou art That."

Immediately the seeker fell into a deep *samadhi*. When he returned to his normal state, he said wonderingly, "But that was exactly what the other Guru told me twelve years ago!"

"Of course," said the Guru. "The Truth hasn't changed in twelve years."

"But why did I have to spend twelve years picking up cow dung?"

"Because your mind was too dense to understand it," said the Guru.

This lovely story is the best introduction I can think of to a book entitled *The Perfect Relationship*. It describes the mysterious simplicity of the Guru-disciple relationship, in which the disciple's obedience and service become the key that unlocks for him the Guru's knowledge. At last, the Guru has only to say a word or two, and the Truth the disciple has been too dull to grasp explodes within him.

In *The Perfect Relationship*, Swami Muktananda touches on all the aspects of the Guru-disciple relationship. As always in his writing, key images and ideas are repeated from chapter to chapter, as if he wanted us to remember that the goal of Siddha Yoga is always the same, and always simple. Swami Muktananda quotes liberally from a wide variety of scriptural texts embracing many traditions, from Vedanta to Kashmir Shaivism. He quotes the poet-saints whose songs were a lifelong source of pleasure to him, especially the great thirteenth century Maharashtran poet, Jnaneshwar. It is as if Swami Muktananda wanted the Siddha tradition itself to speak to us, in all its formidable variety, insisting, century after century, in so many different voices, that the key to Self-realization, the great highway leading to knowledge and love of God, lies in one's longing for the perfect relationship and in the Guru's corresponding role as the soul's "mirror" and the greatest lover.

PAUL ZWEIG
DECEMBER 1980

Definition of Sanskrit Terms

All Sanskrit words, as well as terms that may be unfamiliar to a Western reader, are defined in the Glossary except where an explanation of their meaning is essential to one's understanding of the text. In such cases, they are defined either in the text or in footnotes.

Translation of Devanageri Script

In all quotations, a diacritical mark has been used to indicate the long vowel sounds in Sanskrit, Hindi, and Marathi words. These marks are not used when the same words appear within the body of the text.

The Significance of the Guru

Shri Gurudev is the rising sun of knowledge and expanding intellect. Dwelling on the shore beyond the ocean of discrimination between Self and non-Self, he is the deity who holds the key to the city of liberation and the bliss of the Self. Only one in a thousand people has the desire to know the Self and the Supreme Principle. But when the virtues of many lifetimes have accumulated, one is filled with a burning longing to know That, and this great fortune makes one set out in search of a Guru.

Through the grace of the Sadguru, a person comes to know his own Self and is transformed. Then he makes weeping itself weep and suffering suffer. He raises licentiousness to the lofty position of self-control and forces bad actions and habits to take interest in good ones. His deeds and skills become astonishing. He experiences sense pleasures in renunciation and tastes the bliss of renunciation in sense pleasures. This is the glory of the Guru's grace.

The scriptures and the saints have sung of the Guru's greatness. The great beings say, *gururātmā īshwareti*—"The Guru is the Self as well as God." In the *Yoga Sutras*, Maharishi Patanjali describes God in the aphorism *saha purveshām api guruhu kālenānavachcchedāt*[1]—"Being unconditioned by [space] and time, he is the Guru of all the ancients." The Guru is more ancient than the ancients. The *Guru Gita* also describes the Guru as being identical with God:

brahmānandam parama-sukhadam kevalam jñānamūrtim,
dvandvātītam gagana-sadrusham tattvam asyādilakshyam;
ekam nityam vimalam achalam sarva-dhī-sākshibhūtam,
bhāvātītam triguna-rahitam sadgurum tam namāmi.[2]

---

1. *Patanjali Yoga Sutras*, I, 26.
2. *Guru Gita*, 89.

"I bow to the divine Guru, who is the bliss of the Supreme Absolute, the embodiment of the highest joy, who is supremely independent and the personification of pure knowledge. There is no trace of duality in him. He is perfectly detached and all-pervasive, like the sky. He is the goal of the wisdom of the great statement 'Thou art That.' He is the One without a second. He is eternal, pure, and taintless. He is steady and the witness of all. He is beyond all modifications and devoid of the three *gunas*."[3]

In the great scripture, the *Kularnava Tantra*, it is said, *tataha shrī gururupāyaha sākshāt parāshivāya cha*—"Shri Guru is the means by which Parashiva Himself bestows knowledge." Through the means of Shri Guru, *shaktipat*[4] is bestowed. This process does not originate from a human being, but from God. Therefore, to approach the Guru is to approach God.

Another verse in the *Guru Gita* further explains the significance of the Guru:

dhyānamūlam guror mūrtihi,
pūjāmūlam guroho padam;
mantramūlam guror vākyam,
mokshamūlam guroho krupā.[5]

The first line of this verse is "The root of meditation is the Guru's form." Meditation on a tangible object is superior to meditation on something intangible and imagined, because a person can easily picture in his mind an object that he has already seen. In one of his poems, the great saint Sunderdas writes, *jo mana nārī ke aor nihārat to mana hota hai nārī ke rūpa*[6]—"The mind that contemplates women takes on a woman's form." He goes on to say that just as the mind that

---

3. The *gunas* are the three qualities, *sattva* (purity), *rajas* (activity), and *tamas* (inertia), which interweave to create everything in the universe.
4. The transmission of divine energy, or Shakti; this awakens the recipient's own dormant inner energy, known as Kundalini.
5. *Guru Gita*, 76.
6. *Sundervilas.*

dwells in anger or illusion becomes trapped in anger or illusion, the mind that always contemplates the Guru eventually becomes the Guru. In this way, meditation on the Guru's form immerses the meditator in the state of the Guru. As Patanjali says in one of the aphorisms of the *Yoga Sutras, vītarāga-vishayam vā chittam*[7]—"Focus the mind on one who has risen above passion and attachment." By meditating on a being whose mind is free of attachment and hatred and who has become one with Parabrahman, a person becomes identical with that being.

The second line of the verse is "The root of worship is the Guru's feet." Because the Kundalini Shakti flows continuously from the Guru's feet, it is beneficial to worship and touch them.

The third line is "The root of mantra is the Guru's word." In *Shri Malini Vijaya Tantra* Shiva says, *sa gurur matsamaha prokto mantravīrya prakāshakaha*—"I am that Guru who has made the mantra conscious and who has revealed the potency of the mantra in a disciple." Because the Guru has the power to infuse a mantra with Consciousness, he is the root of the mantra. His word is a mighty mantra.

Finally, "The root of liberation is the Guru's grace." The Guru's compassionate glance is the means to liberation and supreme peace—but the Guru must be a Siddha who has a lineage and who has completely conquered his senses. Without the grace of such a Guru, there is no knowledge and no state of meditation. Without the Guru's company, it is difficult to contemplate the Self. Without the Guru's teaching, there is no discipline in one's life. Without the Guru's blessing, there is no love. Without the Guru's knowledge, there is no end to desire, the intellect does not receive the light of wisdom, the delusion and pain created by duality are not eradicated, nor are doubts dispelled. Happiness and virtue arise from the Guru. When iron comes in contact with the

---

7. *Patanjali Yoga Sutras*, I, 37.

philosophers' stone, it is transmuted into gold. Sandalwood trees infuse their fragrance into the trees around them. In the same way, Shri Gurudev makes a true disciple like himself. This is why it is said:

divya-jnānopadeshtāram deshikam parameshwaram,
pūjayet parayā bhaktyā tasya jnāna-phalam labhet.

"With a feeling of devotion and respect, one should worship as God the Guru who gives the teachings of divine knowledge. Only then can one obtain the fruit of knowledge."

Another text explains the identity of the Guru and God as follows: *brahmavit brahmaiva bhavati*—"One who has known Brahman completely and has merged in Him is Brahman Himself." The *Yogashikopanishad* also states:

yathā gurustathaivesho yathaiveshastathā guruhu,
pūjanīyo mahābhaktyā na bhedo vidyate'nayoho.

"The Guru is God and God is the Guru. Therefore, considering the Guru to be God, one should worship him with all one's heart, with great devotion, respect, and love." The feeling in one's heart draws the Guru's Shakti.

The *Kularnava Tantra* gives many reasons for worshipping the Guru. For example:

gurumūlāha kriyāha sarvā loke'smin kulanāyike,
tasmāt sevyo gurur nityam siddyartham bhakti smayutaihi.[8]

"O Kulanayika, all the yogic *kriyas* in this world arise from the Guru. Therefore, to attain That, one should always serve the Guru with a feeling of devotion." In addition:

brahmā-vishnu-maheshādi devatā-muni-yoginaha,
kurvantyanugraham tushtā gurau tushte na samshayaha.[9]

"When the Guru becomes pleased, Brahma, Vishnu, Mahadeva, and other deities, great seers, and Siddha yogis

---

8. *Kularnava Tantra*, XII, 4.
9. Ibid., XII, 22.

are also pleased and shower blessings. There is no doubt of it." Moreover:

yasya deve parā bhaktir yathā deve tathā gurau,
tasya te kathitā hyarthāha prakāshante kuleshwari.[10]

"O Goddess Kuleshwari, when one has supreme devotion for God and for the Guru, the meaning of the Guru's wisdom reveals itself from within." Then one acquires the capacity to understand the inner mystery.

Another verse in the *Tantra* explains:

guruhu pitā gurur mātā gururdeva maheshwaraha,
shive rushte gurus trātā gurau rushte na kashchana.[11]

"The Guru is the father; the Guru is the mother; the Guru is God. If Shiva is angry the Guru can protect you, but if the Guru becomes angry no one can save you." The Guru is the mother because, like a mother, he always protects his children. The Guru is also the father. There are two kinds of fathers: the physical father, who gives life to a child through his sexual fluid, and the spiritual father, the Guru, who gives life through the mantra. The Guru grants a new birth by bestowing the divine mantra, which contains within it the state of the Self. Through *shaktipat* he gives birth within the seeker to a new, yogic body.

The Guru is perfect in his oneness with Lord Shiva. When God is angry with someone, the Guru protects him. But if the Guru were ever to become angry with anyone, no one would have the power to protect him. The Guru is entirely God.

The *Kularnava Tantra* continues:

guroho shrī pādukā-bhūshā gurunāma smrutir japaha,
gurvājnākaranam krutyam shushrūshā bhajanam guroho.[12]

---

10. Ibid., XII, 33.
11. Ibid., XII, 49.
12. Ibid., XII, 82.

"Shri Guru's feet are the supreme ornaments. To remember the Guru's name is to repeat the mantra. To obey the Guru's command is to perform every kind of good action. To serve the Guru is to sing the divine name." In the same way, repetition with faith, day in and day out, of the mantra given by the Guru is the source of all attainments.

> *guravo bahavah santi dīpavachcha gruhe gruhe,*
> *durlabho'yam gurur devi sūryavat sarvadīpakaha.*[13]

"Every house has a lamp, and in the same way there are many Gurus, but rare is that Guru who, like the sun, gives light to all." Rare is the Guru who, through the inner awakening, makes the light of the Self blaze in everyone's heart.

> *shivo'ham nākrutir devi naradrug gocharo nahi,*
> *tasmāt shrī gururūpena shishyān rakshati dhārmikān.*[14]

"O Goddess! I am Paramashiva. I am Consciousness. [The *Shiva Sutras* say, *chaitanyam ātmā*[15]—"The Self is Consciousness."] I have no form. I cannot be seen by the eyes of human beings. [The *Katha Upanishad* says that the Self is subtler than the subtlest.[16]] Therefore, I enter the Siddha Guru and assume his form. I protect religious people, those who seek happiness, and good disciples."

Not everyone can understand the Guru:

> *shrī gurum paramam tattvam tishthantam chakshuragrataha,*
> *mandabhāgyā na pashyanti hyandhāha sūryamivoditam.*[17]

"Just as the blind cannot see the rising sun, similarly, unfortunate people cannot see the Supreme Principle, Shri Gurudev, even when He is right before their eyes." When one attains true discrimination, one's eye becomes suf-

---

13. Ibid., XIII, 104.
14. Ibid., XIII, 53.
15. *Shiva Sutras*, I, 1.
16. *Katha Upanishad*, I, 2, 20.
17. *Kularnava Tantra*, XII, 15.

ficiently sensitive for one to understand Shri Guru. However, either a guru[18] or a disciple who lacks this discrimination is spiritually blind.

The Qualities of a True Guru

shrī guruhu parameshāni shuddhā-vesho manoharaha,
sarva-lakshana-sampannaha sarvavyava-shobhitaha.[19]

This verse of the *Kularnava Tantra* describes some of the characteristics of Shri Guru. He is clad in spotless clothing, and his bewitching smile reveals that the current of inner bliss flows through all his senses, manifesting outwardly as joy. All his limbs are beautiful and radiate bliss, because the stream of love and the ecstasy and effulgence of the Absolute flow through them. He awakens the Kundalini.

When we first approach a Guru, we should carefully examine his qualities and his actions. He should have conquered desire and anger and banished infatuation from his heart. He should be ecstatic in the intoxication of supreme bliss and virtue. No anguish or agitation should arise in him. The burning of ignorance should have rejected him and passed him by, notions of inequality and disparity should have resigned and left him, and the coolness of supreme peace should have taken up permanent residence within his heart. He should not be attached to anyone because greed, which is the cause of attachment, should have won its freedom from him. He should see no fault in anyone, for his awareness of equality should transform imperfection into perfection and thus make it worthy.

The Guru gives only joy to all; he has banished sorrow. While in the body he has attained liberation, the supreme

---

18. Throughout the book, the word "Guru" is capitalized when it refers to the true Guru and lowercase when it refers to an ordinary teacher.
19. *Kularnava Tantra,* XIII, 38.

state of God. Through him one who is worthy can reach this state instantly; this is known as *nagad dharma*, immediate results. The Guru recognizes the conscious Self everywhere. He harbors no trace of duality and hence has no fear. The great being Sunderdas wrote, "One can never adequately sing the glory of such a Guru." Only such a Guru can truly benefit others; only he is worthy of being called Gurudev.

> *pinda-brahmāndayoraikyam shitam yo vetti tattvataha,*
> *shirāsthi-roma-samkhyādi sa gurur nāparaha priye.*[20]

"O beloved, only that being who is fully aware of the one-ness of the macrocosm and the microcosm and who even knows the number of all the *nadis*, bones, and hairs is in truth a Guru. No one else can be called a Guru."

> *yathā ghatshcha kalashaha kumbhashchaikārtha-vāchakaha,*
> *tathā devashcha mantrashcha gurushchaikārtha uchyate.*[21]

"Just as the three words *ghata, kalasha,* and *kumbha* all mean 'pot,' so are the mantra, the deity of the mantra, and the Guru one and the same." Although God is the One without a second, He manifests as many. A goldsmith may make ornaments in various shapes and with various names, but all are made of gold. In the same way, the One exists in the infinite names and forms of all species. The great saint Jnaneshwar Maharaj wrote that by looking at everything with understanding, a person realizes that the Lord pervades sentient beings, insentient objects, and the world in all its subtle and gross aspects.[22] A person worthy of becoming a Guru is established in this awareness of equality and sees that just as blankets, *dhotis*, shirts, pants, coats, shorts, and so on, are all made from cotton, so also are the mantra, the deity of the mantra, and the Guru one and the same.

The Guru embodies the mantra:

---

20. Ibid., XIII, 88.
21. Ibid., XIII, 64.
22. *Jnaneshwari.*

yathā devastathā mantro yathā mantrastathā guruhu,
devamantragurunām cha pūjayā sadrusha phalam.[23]

"As is the deity, so is the mantra. As is the mantra, so is the
Guru. Therefore, to worship the Guru, the mantra, or the
deity of the mantra with the feeling of service bears the same
fruit." In another text it is also said, *devatā mantrasvarūpinī*—
"The deity is of the form of the mantra."
    Shri Tantra Sadbhava states:

sarve varnātmakā mantrāste cha shaktyātmakāha priye,
shaktistu mātrukā jneyā sa cha jneyā shivātmikā.

"O dear one, all mantras consist of letters. The letters are
forms of Shakti. That Shakti is known as *matruka,* and
matruka is the very form of Shiva." In this way, the mantra,
the Guru, and the deity of the mantra are completely one.
    In *Jnaneshwari,*[24] the commentary on the *Bhagavad Gita* by
Jnaneshwar Maharaj, the Lord says, "When true knowledge
arises in a person's heart, I become the Vedas for him in the
form of inner knowledge. In the form of mantras, I help him
to perform fire rituals and other actions. I assume the form of
the Guru to give a seeker the knowledge of My own Self."
Similarly, the Lord says in the *Kularnava Tantra:*

shivarūpam samāsthāya pūjām gruhnāmi pārvati,
gururūpam samādāya bhavapāshānnikruntaye.[25]

"O Parvati! Assuming the form of Shiva, I accept all worship;
assuming the form of the Guru, I cut the noose of worldliness." Shiva, the primordial Guru, further states:

siddhānta-sāra vettāham bījo'hamiti bodhakrut,
avichchhinnaha sadā hrushtahrudayo gurur uchyate.[26]

---

23. *Kularnava Tantra,* XIII, 65.
24. Jnaneshwar's commentary on the *Bhagavad Gita* takes the form of an
amplification of the original dialogue between Krishna and Arjuna in which
Jnaneshwar assumes the voices of the speakers.
25. *Kularnava Tantra,* XIII, 66.
26. Ibid., XIII, 67.

"Dwelling in everyone's heart as the witness, I know the essence of all doctrines. I am the seed of the world. As the Guru, I am eternal and the giver of knowledge." According to another scripture, *tathā hridaya-bījasya vishvam etat charā-charam*—"The seed of the entire world of insentient objects and sentient beings is in His heart." In the *Bhagavad Gita* the Lord says, *bhoktā maheshwara*, which means that in the form of individuals, He is the experiencer of all. Thus, the Guru is both the conscious power that bestows knowledge and the Self.

A true Guru is not trapped in anything, nor is he concealed. He has risen above both body and senses. With the coolness of imperishable peace and knowledge, he puts differences to flight. Through his perfection and his pure awareness of the all-pervasive and perfect Absolute, he roots out impure thoughts. Viewing everything as equal, he destroys the sense of duality and the other impediments to the perception of God's unity. In the fire of the knowledge of unity, he consumes all the doubts that create duality and make one burn in agitation, jealousy, negligence, and desire. To one who wants peace, he gives the natural, sublime, and auspicious two-syllabled mantra *so'ham*. I offer my salutations to that indivisible Guru.

The Guru should possess every virtue. A person who lacks renunciation, purity, good conduct, virtue, unwavering knowledge of the Absolute, the wisdom of yoga, or devotion can never be a Guru. He cannot be a true Guru if he engages in business, in different material pursuits or therapies, if he supports dancing and the use of marijuana, opium, and other intoxicants, or if he indulges in sense pleasures. A disciple who discovers such behavior in a guru can only benefit by considering him a worm of bad conduct and rejecting him.

One morning, Guru Bhagawan Sheik Sahib was giving a lecture in a coffeehouse. The room was crowded because the price of admission was very low. The *sheik* began to speak about high knowledge, true religion, and perfect teachings. He said, "All Gurus except me are false. Only I am perfect and true. No one has attained as much knowledge as I have, and no one has ever taught this kind of knowledge. Be happy and behave in whatever way you like."

After he had given this teaching, he said, "Now I am going to give you my final instructions. It is wicked to smoke cigarettes, so give them up. It is wrong to drink liquor. Moreover, you should not spend time with women unnecessarily." With these words, he concluded his lecture and then added, "If anyone wants to ask a question, he may do so."

One man stood up and said, "O Sheik, there is a pack of cigarettes in your pocket!"

The *sheik* replied, "Yes, I smoke."

A second man said, "O Sheik Sahib, I always see you drinking liquor in bars."

"Oh, yes. It's my daily practice."

Another said, "I see you walking around the park with a different woman every day."

"Yes, of course I do that."

"Then what were you talking about at the end of your lecture?"

"I was just imparting knowledge to you," Sheik Sahib said. "I don't follow it myself."

One cannot obtain strength from such gurus. A Sadguru should be like a supremely holy place of pilgrimage.

A true Guru is proficient at distinguishing between that which is correct and that which is incorrect according to scriptural doctrines. One can perceive the Supreme Principle through his mere gesture. By hearing him speak, one is freed from delusion and doubts and can understand even the most difficult subject. Only such a superior being is a Guru worthy of giving *shaktipat* initiation and knowledge of the Truth.

antar lakshyo bahir drushtihi sarvajno deshakālavit,
ājnāsiddhis trikālajno nigrahānugraha-kshamaha.[27]

"Although his eyes appear to look outside, his gaze is constantly fixed on the inner Self. He is omniscient, and supernatural powers follow him. He knows space and time, past, present, and future. If he commands someone to do something, it always bears fruit. He is able to bestow grace and mete out punishment." Only such a superior person is worthy of being called a Guru.

vedhako bodhakaha shāntaha sarvajīva-dayākaraha,
svādhīnendriya-sanchāra shad-varga-vijayapradaha.[28]

"He can pierce the *chakras*. He gives one the wisdom of Siddha Yoga. He is serene and bestows compassion on all people. He moves through the world with his senses under control. He has conquered the six enemies."[29] Through the power of the Self, the Guru transmits his Shakti into others. Only such a compassionate Guru can uplift his disciples.

agraganyo 'tigambhīraha pātrāpātra visheshavit,
shiva-vishnu-samaha sādhu-manu-bhūshanabhūshitaha.[30]

"He is foremost among all. He is profound and can distinguish between the worthy and the unworthy. He is like Shiva and Vishnu. Noble and wise people are his ornaments. He is proficient in all actions." He has assimilated Siddha Yoga and attained the fearlessness of the Self. He regards all deities and religions as equal. Only such an incomparable being is a Guru.

nirmamo nitya-santushtaha svatantro'nantashaktimān,
sadbhakta-vatsalo dhīraha krupāluhu smitapūrnavāk.[31]

---

27. Ibid., XIII, 41.
28. Ibid., XIII, 42.
29. The six enemies are desire, greed, anger, lust, envy, and infatuation.
30. *Kularnava Tantra*, XIII, 43.
31. Ibid., XIII, 44.

"He is free of attachment. He is always happy and independent. He has infinite powers. He has affection for good devotees. He is brave and compassionate. He is always smiling, and his speech brings joy." Only one who possesses these qualities can be a Guru.

svavidyānushthāna-rato-dharma-jnānārtha-darshakaha,
yadruchchhā-lābha-santushto guna-dosha-vibhedakaha.[32]

"Such a one is engaged in the pursuit of knowledge [and meditation]. He reveals the meaning of wisdom and righteousness. He can explain the difference between good and evil. He remains satisfied with whatever comes to him through God's will." Only such a superior person is a Guru worthy of initiating disciples into knowledge of the Absolute.

In the *Bhagavad Gita* is the following description of an enlightened being:

udāsīnavadāsīno gunair yo na vichālyate,
gunā vartanta ityeva yo'vatishthati nengate.[33]

"Seated like one unconcerned, he is not controlled by the *gunas*. Knowing that the *gunas* are active, he is centered in his own Self and does not move." In Jnaneshwar's commentary on this verse, Krishna tells Arjuna:

"Knowing that all the *gunas* operate of their own accord and exist because of the Self, he does not fall into the trap of analyzing or discussing them. Possessing this complete knowledge, he takes shelter in the body like a traveler who stays for a while at a guest house. Like a battlefield, which neither wins a victory nor suffers defeat, he does not share in gain or loss. He neither involves himself with the *gunas* nor is affected by them. Just as the *prana* is in the body, yet remains different from it, an enlightened being is indif-

---

32. Ibid., XIII, 47.
33. *Bhagavad Gita*, XIV, 23.

ferent to his physical body. He lives in it while inwardly remaining completely fulfilled by perfect love and bliss. O Arjuna, just as Mount Meru is not disturbed by the waves of a mirage, an enlightened being is not annoyed by the *gunas*. The sky cannot be shaken by the wind, darkness cannot hide the sun, nor can dreams deceive a person who is awake. Similarly, the *gunas* cannot bind an enlightened being. He never falls into their clutches, but calmly observes them from afar, just as a spectator in a theater quietly watches a puppet show.

"This is the state of an enlightened being. By the light of the sun, all people carry out their activities and deeds, yet the sun remains motionless and watches everything. Whether the wind blows forcefully or very gently, the sky remains unmoved and motionless. In the same way, an enlightened being remains unperturbed even when he comes in contact with the *gunas*."[34]

Only a being who lives in this state can be a Guru. The *Kularnava Tantra* says:

tulya-nindāstutir maunī nirāpeksho niyāmakaha,
ityādi-lakshanopetaha shrī guruhu kathitaha priye. [35]

"O beloved, he is called a Guru who has such qualities as serenity, desirelessness, self-control, and equanimity in the face of praise and censure." Thus, the Guru is wise and detached and has realized the Self through the Siddha Path. He does not indulge in sense pleasures. He neither keeps bad company nor becomes ensnared in addictions. He is free of conflicts, desires, and thoughts. He is disciplined and possesses self-control, and he also makes his disciples observe discipline. He is very tender, sweet, and impartial. He carries on no business other than the duties of Guruhood. He places praise and blame on the same seat, regarding them as

---

34. *Jnaneshwari,* XIV, 334-358.
35. *Kularnava Tantra,* XIII, 50.

equal, and he always contemplates the Supreme Truth. A person who possesses all these virtues is worthy of being a Guru, of giving initiation into Siddha Yoga, and of granting the knowledge of the Self.

In India, only perfect Gurus are given the highest respect. The lineage of Gurus is very long. There have been countless sages, seers, and yogis of great power whose lineage remains alive and who continue to carry out their work in this world from time to time. When the selection of one who is to become a Guru is supported by the full grace of the Siddhas, a Siddha Guru gives him the command to serve others and confers Guruhood upon him. When a Guru's mission in his present incarnation comes to an end, he summons his disciple and transfers into his heart that which he has in his own. Sometimes, through the full grace of his Guru, a disciple reaches the state of perfection while the Guru is still alive. The great Siddha Gahininath bestowed his full grace on Nivrittinath while still living, and Nivrittinath in turn gave his full grace to Jnaneshwar Maharaj during his own lifetime. While Guru Janardan Swami was living, he conferred his full grace on Ekanath Maharaj. A Siddha Guru prepares a disciple for a long time, testing him in many ways and thus freeing him from all faults. Only then does he command the disciple to become a Guru. These tests are meant only for those who are to become Gurus. Otherwise, a Siddha Guru can give supreme bliss, the experience of the Self, and liberation in this lifetime to anyone, and no difficult tests are necessary. Through a Siddha Guru's grace alone, many individuals are liberated. The Guru makes a worldly person recognize his own Self through the knowledge of meditation; his compassion is the means by which ordinary people cross over the world.

Sunderdas wrote, "Through the Guru's grace, an evil intellect becomes good and turns toward the light of the Self. Through the blessing of the Guru's knowledge and Shakti, I have completely forgotten the unremitting pain of worldliness. The love that the entire world seeks in one thing or another I found within myself through the Guru's grace. Through his grace, I received the blissful name of God, which grants all attainments. Through his grace, I easily acquired the skills of yoga. Through the grace of Shri Guru, I gained equanimity of mind and the state of *samadhi* in the Supreme Void. Sunderdas says that whoever receives Guru-dev's grace easily attains the knowledge of the Truth."[36]

The Lineage

Lord Shiva is the source of Guruhood.

jagadguru namas tubhyam shivāya shivadāya cha,
yogīndrānām cha yogīndra gurunām gurava namaha.

Using mantras such as those in the verse above, all deities, sages, and seers have addressed Lord Shankara as the Guru of the entire world, the Lord of yogis, and the Guru of Gurus.

The supreme knowledge of Siddha Yoga first manifested from the effulgence of Shiva and the form of Shakti, the supreme energy. It arose from the body of Uma Kumari,[37] God's power of will. (The *Shiva Sutras* say, *ichchāshaktir umā kumārī*[38]—"The power of will is the maiden Uma.") For this reason, without the grace of yogini Kundalini, the great Shakti, the supreme state is difficult to attain. This Shakti of the *maha* yoga is the basis of everything. She is Consciousness.

The *Maha Yoga Vijnana*,[39] a great text of Siddha Yoga, explains how the Siddha Yoga lineage originated with Para-shiva and was passed on to Lord Narayana, who assumed

---

36. *Sundervilas.*
37. Uma is a name for the consort of Shiva.
38. *Shiva Sutras,* I, 13.
39. A compilation of Sanskrit verses from various scriptures, with explanations in Hindi by Bramachari Yogananda of Hrishikesh.

the form of a yogi and taught Siddha Yoga to all the sages. After this, the great sage Bhagawan Sanatkumara gave the wisdom of this sublime yoga to Samvarta, the best among sages. The great yogi Sanandana granted it to the sage Pulaha, and he in turn gave it to the sage Gautama. The sage Angiras gave it to the seer Bharadwaja, the knower of the Vedas. The Siddha Kapilamuni, the king of yogis, conferred the same knowledge on the yogi Jaigishavya as well as on Panchashikhacharya.

In the *Kurma Purana*,[40] the great sage Bhagawan Vedavyasa explained how Shri Maheshwar and other sages and seers passed on Siddha Yoga from one to another, imbibing it while continuing to perform all their duties. Speaking to a great assemblage of sages, he told how his father, the sage Parashara, who was a knower of all the principles of manifestation, received this supreme knowledge from Yogindra Bhagawan Sanakamuni and passed it on to Valmiki, author of the *Ramayana*. Then Bhagawan Vedavyasa, the best of sages and Narayan incarnate, related how the great yogi Bhagawan Vamadeva (who had assumed the form of Rudra holding a bow in his hand) taught this knowledge to him. He said that when he received the highest knowledge of this great yoga from Rudravamadeva, supreme devotion for Shankara arose in him. He then exhorted everyone to take refuge in Supreme Shiva, Shankara, Trishuli, who is a haven for those who turn to Him. When he finished speaking, he and all the sages offered their thanks to Shankara, proclaiming that through His grace they had attained Shakti, supreme love, and devotion to Shri Guru Shiva, who has taken the form of the universe and is the Self of all. Then the sages bowed with humility and declared that repetition of the name of Supreme Shiva, the mantra *om namah shivaya*, is the highest devotion to Him. Finally, having explained that this mantra is difficult even for celestial beings to obtain, all the sages returned to their respective places.

---

40. *Kurma Purana*, II, 11.

The Characteristics of a False Guru

So far we have examined some of the characteristics of Shri Guru. It is also important to understand something about those who assume the position of the Guru without having had a Guru, without having reached the state of Guruhood, without having received the command of a Guru, and without having attained the Truth. One who wears the clothes of a Guru without knowing the Truth can easily take simple, straightforward people in the wrong direction. Because so many have been misled by false gurus, the world has developed a new hatred even for supremely pure Gurus.

The characteristics of a false guru are described in the third chapter of the *Kamaksha Tantra*:

samskāra-rahito mūrkho veda-shāstra-vivarjitaha,
shrauta-smārta-kriyā-shūnyaha
shushka-bhāshaha sukutsitaha.[41]

This verse states that a false guru has not been initiated through the rites of any sacred ceremony. He is a fool and lacks the knowledge of the Vedic scriptures. He does not have a sacred thread or tuft, nor has he taken proper *sannyasa*. He does not observe the practices laid down in the scriptures, such as bathing, meditation, and the regular recitation of scriptural texts. He neither knows the disciplines of yoga nor performs them. His words are meaningless, and he condemns others.

pura-yājana-jīvī cha naro vaidyashcha kāmukaha,
krūro dambhī matsarī cha vyasanī krupanaha khalaha.[42]

"He is a man who lives by performing rituals. He is a giver of medicines. He is passionate, cruel, hypocritical, jealous, a slave to addictions, miserly, and a cheat." He attains the position of guru by displaying magic or attracts people by giving them herbs, roots, or other medicine. (Today there are

---

41. *Kamaksha Tantra*, III, 2; quoted in *Maha Yoga Vijnana*.
42. Ibid., III, 3.

many gurus who draw people by giving out medicine or drugs.) He dons the clothing of a holy man, sets himself up as a guru, and imparts teachings. He indulges himself completely in sense pleasures. He overeats. He is by nature harsh and pretentious. To obtain fame and money, he performs actions prohibited by the scriptures. He engages people in worldly pleasures and deceit, and makes corruption flourish. He tells lies, behaves shamelessly, and is a cunning swindler. Sooner or later, the boat of such a guru will sink.

kusangī nāstiko bhīto mahāpātaka-chinhitaha. [43]

"He keeps bad company. He is an atheist, is fearful, and has the characteristics of a great sinner." Such a guru merely seeks to profit from his disciples. He makes them behave licentiously. He deals in drugs and attempts to lead people into meditation by giving them marijuana, opium, and cocaine. He himself is addicted to intoxicants. He is miserly, wicked, and bestial and does evil to others. He is a gossip, and because of actions that he performed in his past lives or in his present lifetime, he has developed hemorrhoids, corns, and skin discoloration and has contracted stomach diseases, dysentery, asthma, and tuberculosis. Because his body has lost its sexual fluid, it reeks. He is indebted to many people. He has become a mental case. A seeker should not forget himself in astonishment when such a guru displays drugs and supernatural powers. Such a being can never be a giver of liberation, for he is utterly false. One who continually begs and borrows from his disciples can never be a Sadguru.

The Burden of Worldly Life

One should courageously try to know one's own Self through meditation. A person who is ignorant of the Self is

---

43. Ibid., III, 4.

always troubled. All his life, he keeps shifting his pain from one shoulder to the other. A woman tires of her husband; a man tires of his wife. One person exhausts himself thinking about a second marriage, and another becomes tired of his business. A third considers changing his profession but finally puts himself in the hands of a psychologist. A human being is always caught up in his desires. Chasing after them, he exchanges one kind of pain for another, but he never changes himself. Day in and day out, there is only fatigue in his life—no meditation, no prayer, no chanting of God's name, no knowledge of the Self, no awareness that his life is flying by in vain. He goes from sorrow to sorrow, but he does not root out the source of the pain. No matter how much he suffers, he remains completely absorbed in his worldly life.

In this way, a person passes through his life until death finally appears before him. At the moment of his death, he has a vision of his life and realizes that it has been a mountain of suffering. Then, terrified of dying, he loses his courage. After so many years of engaging his body, his mind, his whole life in suffering, he has earned only fear. This is the reward for his arduous striving, the fruit of his lifelong craving for joy. This is what he has attained as a result of his ever-present and limitless desires.

When Lord Buddha saw the suffering of the world, he said, "All that I see in this world is birth and death. Death follows birth, disease follows health, old age follows youth. As one watches this pain and constant suffering, one ultimately sees that there are only faults in the world and becomes afraid of it." The *Bhagavad Gita* describes this understanding as *janma-mrityu-jarā-vyādhi-duhkha-doshānudarshanam*[44]—"perception of the evil of birth, death, old age, sickness, and pain." To have this perception is the greatest of all worldly attainments. When Lord Buddha began to see the world in this way, he decided to relinquish his kingdom; he

---

44. *Bhagavad Gita*, XIII, 8.

was convinced that there could not be any more suffering in the forest than on the throne. With this understanding, he left his palace accompanied by Channa, the keeper of the royal stables, who was an ordinary man of the world. When they reached the forest, Lord Buddha ordered Channa to leave. Channa pleaded, "O prince, do not do this. You are still a young man. You have had no experience of life. Do not run away out of fear of the world. Do not give up your kingdom. There is so much joy in life! You are a prince—you have elephants, horses, wealth! Where will you go after giving these up? Even a poor, small man like me is not ready to leave this life, and you are a sovereign. Turn around and look at your kingdom! What do you lack?"

Lord Buddha looked back and then said to Channa, "I see nothing there except pain and intrigue. I have thoroughly experienced the palace life and the activities of the kingdom which appear to be so joyful to you. To you they are a show, but to me they are a source of pain. That which seems pleasurable to you has brought only sorrow to me. Suffering is hidden behind the face of pleasure. Channa, return!"

There is pain in a poor man's life; his poverty is the means by which he hides the true source of his suffering. Similarly, anguish lies beneath the ostentatious wealth of a rich man, who displays riches in order to disguise his pain. In the course of their lives people often greet pain in silence. One person conceals his torment in a hut and another in a palace; one hides it in a solitary place and another among people. But suffering is the same everywhere.

What is the source of this pain? We experience it because we beg for happiness where it does not exist; instead of wanting that which is right for us, we seek that which we can never attain. We desire to make the impossible possible. This world is like a boardinghouse or a Hilton Hotel in which we are temporary guests. Trying to find eternity here is like trying to stop a river whose very nature is to flow. We seek outer love, which is transitory. We want that love to be undying, but how can we attain undying love from something ephemeral? In fact, if we consider this matter with understanding, we will realize that we experience our greatest suffering in the name of love. *Hruddeshe 'rjuna tishthati*[45]—"God dwells in the heart." But although God, the embodiment of love, resides within us, most people are so unfortunate that they do not see love even in their dreams. Even a person who has labored all his life to attain love is unhappy; in the name of love, he experiences only pain. Without true love, everyone suffers—renunciants, sensualists, those who have great wealth, and those who have nothing. A poor person suffers because he has no wealth. A rich person suffers because he has too much wealth. You may look for a truly happy person, but you will never find one.

You will attain happiness only if you stand firmly in the face of the anguish that you encounter. Do not run from it. Look pain squarely in the face; then you will understand it. Know that without knowledge or meditation, without discovering the inspiration of the Self, you will experience only heartache and the misery of living without love for God. Without meditation, life is filled with sorrow. Without the bliss of the Self, there is unquestionably nothing but suffering.

Lord Buddha said, "A life without knowledge is painful." Old age and death are miserable when one lacks knowledge of the Self. In fact, without this knowledge, all of life—from one corner to the other, from east to west, from north to south, above and below—is filled with anguish.

The Path to Freedom

The sages and saints have said that to end suffering and attain happiness, one must have knowledge of the Self, which is the true source of joy. *Jnānam tu parama-gatihi—*

---

45. Ibid., XVIII, 61.

"Knowledge is the supreme state." The bliss of the Self is attained only through knowledge. In the *Bhagavad Gita* the Lord says, *na hi jnānena sadrusham pavitramiha vidyate*[46]— "In this world, there is nothing as pure as knowledge."

Bhāve hi vidyate devo—"God exists in one's feeling." There is great power in a person's feeling. Through it he can make God manifest. Because his feeling is the result of his understanding, right understanding is the source of all attainments, mundane as well as spiritual. *Jnānādeva tu kaivalyam*—"The supreme state comes only from knowledge." Through knowledge a wise person turns poison into nectar: Mirabai drank poison, considering it God's nectar, and was unaffected by it. But through his nonawareness, an ignorant person turns nectar into poison. The truth is that there is neither nectar in nectar nor poison in poison. Everything depends on one's attitude and understanding. For a person who has the supreme knowledge of God's all-pervasiveness, even a dark forest is a celestial garden and even a prison is a wide-open space. But for one who does not know his own Self, who does not regard others as himself, even a celestial garden is like a prison.

That is why it does not matter where you are or where you live, but rather who you are and what your inner state happens to be. The problem lies in your ignorance of your own essential nature. You will gain nothing by changing your country, town, or home; since you take your own destiny with you, you will only be welcoming pain again. It is very good to want freedom, but instead of looking for it in the wrong place, you must discover where it really dwells. The difference between a spiritual being and a politician is this: The politician says, "Bondage is external—break it and then you will obtain the joy of freedom." But the knower of the Truth says, "O my friend, bondage is not outside, but within you." No matter how much you try to break your

---

46. Ibid., IV, 38.

outer fetters, your bondage will only increase. Therefore, you must go where there is supreme freedom—to the inner Self in the heart.

You are entirely responsible for your own state of dependency; in fact, you have become addicted to it. Because you think that the elixir of love is found in dependency, you have made it the abode of your love, and if you were ever to tear down the wall of dependency, you would only build another one somewhere else. However, you must free yourself in every way. Lord Buddha said again and again, "You can certainly come to me, but do not become bound by me." In the same way, when people ask me, "Is it alright to meditate on you?" I tell them, "Meditate on your own Self." Although it is difficult, you must escape from the prison of the non-Self. Who is a Hindu? Who is a Vaishnavite? Who is a Jain, a Buddhist, a Sufi, or a Christian? If you are imprisoned in one of these false identities, how can you find the freedom of the Self? That is why Lord Krishna said, *sarvadharmān partiyajya māmekam sharanam vraja*[47]—"Give up all religions and take refuge in Me alone." Discard all false identification with religion. Go to the inner Self for shelter and revel there.

The Power of Grace

It is true that *jīvo brahmaiva nāparaha*—"The individual soul is nothing but God." Still, in order for one to have the full experience of the Self as Consciousness, the Guru is as necessary as *prana*, the life force, is necessary to the body. The body without *prana* is desolate; in the same way, life without the Guru is dry.

According to Kashmir Shaivism, *gururupāyaha*[48]—"The

---

47. Ibid., XVIII, 66.
48. *Shiva Sutras*, II, 6.

Guru is the means." Through the Guru, one attains the power of the Self. The word "Guru" has two syllables: *gu* and *ru*. *Gukārastvandhakārashcha rukārasteja uchyate*[49]—"*Gu* means darkness and *ru* means light." *Gu* represents the darkness which envelops the Self, and *ru* represents that principle which destroys the darkness of ignorance and reveals the light of wisdom. It is the Guru who gives knowledge of the Supreme Principle. The *Shiva Sutras* also say that the Guru is the means of attaining *mantra virya* and *mudra virya*. *Mantra virya* is the experience of *purno'ham*, the perfect "I"-consciousness, the seed of all. *Mudra virya* is the *khechari mudra*, the state of Supreme Bhairava. One who experiences these attains eternal peace; the supreme state is reached when lack of peace, which arises from dualistic awareness, no longer exists.

It is important to understand that the Guru is not merely a human being but an eternal principle, the power of grace. A Shaivite text says, *guror gurutarā shaktir guruvaktragata bhavet*[50]—"The power of the Guru's grace inherent in his speech is greater than the Guru himself." Moreover, even though this power of grace is transmitted from one Guru to another, it is actually the power of God; in his commentary on the *Shiva Sutras*, Kshemaraja writes, *gurur vā pārameshwarī anugrāhikā shaktihi*[51]—"The Guru is the grace-bestowing power of God." The bestowal of grace is one of the five functions of God, and because the Guru is the being in whom God's power resides, he is worshipped as God.

Shiva said, *sa gurur matsamaha prokto mantravīryaprakāshakaha*[52]—"That Guru who reveals the potency of the mantra is just like Me." A Guru causes the knowledge of *aham brahmāsmi*—"I am the Absolute"—to arise. It is the Guru's Shakti, rather than the individual, which is the

---

49. *Guru Gita*, 46.
50. *Mantrishivobhairava*.
51. Kshemaraja, *Shiva Sutra Vimarshini*.
52. *Shri Malini Vijaya Tantra*, II, 10.

Guru. That Shakti is transmitted by the Guru, awakens the disciple's own inner Shakti, called Kundalini, and thus gives the disciple the experience of the expansion of consciousness. The Shakti is infinite and perfect. It bestows the experience of the oneness of the individual soul and Shiva, and makes one revel continually in the bliss of the Self. *Santoshādanuttama-sukhalābhaha*[53]—"When one becomes established in contentment, one attains extraordinary happiness."

Through the Guru's grace, desire and futile hopes are destroyed. When the mind becomes free of desire, one experiences bliss. No other joy can be likened to this inner bliss; even the joy of heaven is infinitesimal by comparison.

How is this happiness attained? One of the aphorisms in the *Pratyabhijnahridayam* is *madhya-vikāsāt chidānanda-lābhaha*[54]—"The unfoldment of the central *nadi* [subtle channel] gives rise to the bliss of Consciousness." The *madhya nadi* is the *sushumna*. The *Prashnopanishad* explains the *nadis* as follows:

hrudi hyesha ātmā, atraitad ekashatam nādinām,
tāsām shatam shatam ekaikasyām, dvāsaptatir dvāsaptatihi,
pratishākhā-nādī, sahasrāni bhavantyāsu vyānashcharati.[55]

"The seat of the individual soul is the heart region. [The *Bhagavad Gita* says the same thing: *hruddeshe'rjuna tishthati*.] There are one hundred *nadis* in the heart. From each of these *nadis*, seventy-two additional *nadis* branch out. And again, each of these *nadis* has one thousand sub-branches. Thus, there are 720 million *nadis*, through which the vital air called *vyana* flows."

The central *nadi*, the *sushumna*, is the primary basis and source of all the other *nadis*. The unfoldment of the central

---

53. *Patanjali Yoga Sutras*, II, 42.
54. Kshemaraja, *Pratyabhijnahridayam*, 18.
55. *Prashnopanishad*, III, 6.

nadi signifies the blossoming of one's fortune. This takes place automatically once the Kundalini is awakened.

> *āmūladhārād ābrahmabilam vilasantim,*
> *bisatantu-tanīyasim vidyut-punja-pinjarām,*
> *vivasvad-ayutabhāsvat prakāshām parām,*
> *shata-sudhā-mayukha-shitala-tejo-danda-rūpam,*
> *parachitim kundalinīm bhāvayet.*[56]

"Contemplate Kundalini, who is Supreme Consciousness, who plays from the *muladhara* to the *sahasrara*, who shines like a flash of lightning, who is as fine as a fiber of a lotus stalk, who has the brilliant radiance of countless suns, and who is a shaft of light as cool as hundreds of nectarean moonbeams." Chitshakti, God's power of Universal Consciousness, extends from the *muladhara*, the spiritual center at the base of the spine, to the *sahasrara*, the spiritual center at the crown of the head. She is very subtle and shines like a flash of lightning. She has the form of the light of countless rays of the sun and moon. She pervades the entire body. When one becomes worthy of receiving Her grace, She is awakened through the grace of the Guru. Then meditation takes place automatically, and a spontaneous inner yoga is activated; when the all-pervasive Chitshakti unfolds in the central *nadi*, the process of yoga occurs spontaneously in all the *nadis*. Ultimately, the great Shakti brings Siddha Yoga to its completion and makes one merge into Shiva. For the awakening of Kundalini, the grace of Shri Guru is essential. Therefore, the Guru's grace is an integral part of Siddha Yoga.

The Disciple

We have examined the characteristics of the Guru, the path shown by the Guru, and some of the effects of the Guru's

---

56. *Shri Vidya Antar Yaga.*

grace. Now let us look at the recipient of that grace, the disciple. Like the Sadguru, a worthy disciple has specific characteristics.

First, however, let us examine the qualities of a false disciple. In the *Kularnava Tantra*, Shiva describes him in this way:

dushta-vamshodbhavam dushtam gunahīnam virūpinam,
parashishyam cha pāshandam shandam panditamāninam.[57]

"He is wicked, lacks virtues, and comes from a corrupt family. He is a heretic and takes pride only in dry and scholarly knowledge. He becomes the disciple of any teacher he encounters." He performs bad actions, is given to self-praise, and lacks perfection.

utsrushtam durmukham chāpi svechchha-veshadharam param,
durvikārānga-cheshtādi gatibhāshana-bhīshanam.[58]

"He is shunned by the members of his family and by society. His parents, fellow townsmen, and Guru reject him. The mere sight of him creates fear. He is foul-mouthed. He dresses in whatever way he likes. [This does not apply to actors and actresses.]" Sometimes he becomes a *sadhu;* at other times he tosses aside his *sadhu* clothing and gets a job. He takes the great initiation of *sannyasa,* and then gets married and falls from his vows. His speech creates restlessness and fear.

After listing the characteristics of a false disciple, Mahadev describes the qualities of a good, pure, fortunate, and virtuous disciple:

sachchhishyam tu kuleshāni shubha-lakshana-samyutam,
samādhi-sādhanopetam guna-shīla-samanvitam.[59]

". . . He is engaged in the *sadhana* leading to *samadhi* [*yama,*

---

57. *Kularnava Tantra*, XIII, 3.
58. Ibid., XIII, 5.
59. Ibid., XIII, 23.

niyama, asana, the techniques of hatha yoga, natural *prana-yama,* and so on]. He is endowed with noble qualities. He is good-natured and behaves correctly." He is worthy of receiving Shakti and the knowledge of the Truth.

> *svachchha-dehāmbaram prājnam dhārmikam*
> *shuddha-mānāsam,*
> *dridha-vritam sadāchāram shraddhābhakti-samanvitam.*[60]

"He has a pure mind and is gifted with faith and devotion. He knows the scriptures. He is endowed with a beautiful body and wears clean clothes. He observes good conduct." Such a disciple is deserving of initiation.

> *dakshamalpāshinam gūdhachittam nirvyāja-sevakam,*
> *vimrushyakārinam vīram manodāridrya-varjitam.*[61]

"He performs actions with understanding and with unselfish motives. He has a generous mind and is a profound thinker. He eats sparingly. He is careful and competent in his actions. He is courageous and free of pride." Such a noble person is qualified for initiation.

> *sarvakāryāti-kushalam svachchham sarvopakārinam,*
> *krutājnām pāpabhītancha sādhu-sajjana-sammatam.*[62]

"He carries out all his actions with great skill. He finds joy in helping others. He is pure because of his virtuous actions and is afraid to perform sinful deeds. He is grateful and assimilates the qualities of noble people." Such a person is regarded as a superior disciple and is closely related to the Guru.

> *āstikam dāna-shīlam cha sarva-bhūta-hite-ratam,*
> *vishvāsa-vinayopetam dhana-dedādya-vanchakam.*[63]

---

60. Ibid., XIII, 24.
61. Ibid., XIII, 25.
62. Ibid., XIII, 26.
63. Ibid., XIII, 27.

"He is a staunch believer. He is charitable and is engaged in service to others. He never deceives people or takes away their money. He is worthy of the Guru's trust. He is humble, egoless, free of pride, and always happy." Such a person is a worthy disciple.

asādhya-sādhakam shūram utsāha-bala-samyutam,
anukūla-kriyā yuktam apramattam vichakshanam.[64]

"He is a wise person who, through *sadhana* and the power of his enthusiasm, makes possible that which is impossible. He never neglects to engage himself in austerities and suitable work. He is courageous." Such a person is worthy of receiving the knowledge of the Absolute.

hita-satya-mita-smera-bhāshanām muktadūshanam,
sakrudukta-gruhītārtham chaturam buddhi-vistaram.[65]

"His speech is beneficial to others, true, and pure. It always brings joy. He speaks little. He is very intelligent and sharp-witted. When he is told something once, he understands it." Such an intelligent disciple is the child of the Guru and is qualified to receive the knowledge of the Absolute.

svastutau paranindāyām vimukham sumukham priye,
jitendriyam susantushtam dhīmantam brahmachārinam.[66]

"He dislikes hearing himself praised and others criticized. He is always pleased and eager to do for others work that is important to them. He has mastered his senses and is disciplined in his actions."

He regards the Guru as the Self. He considers his vital force to be the Guru and his body to be the disciple. By imbibing the Guru's wisdom, he has become the Guru, yet he never forgets his own discipleship. Such a disciple is the child of the Guru and is worthy of receiving initiation into yoga.

---

64. Ibid., XIII, 28.
65. Ibid., XIII, 29.
66. Ibid., XIII, 30.

guru-daivata-sambhaktam kāmini-pūjakam param,
nityam gurusamīpastham guru-santoshā-kārakam.[67]

"He always remains close to the Guru and does that work
which pleases the Guru. Through meditation he worships the
great Shakti Kundalini, the Goddess and mother of the world.
He has complete devotion to the Guru and the deity." Such a
person is worthy of receiving supreme initiation; between him
and the Guru there exists the relationship of father and child.

A true disciple nurtures the secret knowledge taught by the
Guru, and never disobeys the Guru's command. Because he
considers the Guru to be Shiva, all attainments come to him
on their own.

*Yo guruhu saha shiva yo shivaha saha guru ubhayorantam nāsti
shabdiararthai*—"The Guru is Shiva and Shiva is the Guru.
There is no difference between them, other than words."
There is a sublime relationship between a Guru and a disciple
who has this awareness.

Once a disciple named Gahini went in search of the great
Guru Gorakhnath. He met the Guru on the road and immediately fell at his feet. Gorakhnath said, "Sit here. I'll be
back." He left Gahini sitting at the side of the road and returned twelve years later. By that time Gahini was already a
full Siddha. Gorakhnath said to him, "Go! You are complete.
Follow the discipline and ways of the Naths. Teach true disciples." The same Gahininath became the Guru of Nivrittinath,
who was the Guru of Jnaneshwar Maharaj.

Nivrittinath taught meditation and chanting. It was his
experience that chanting prepared a person for *shaktipat* and
made the Shakti rise. He said:

ugavale bimba advaita svayambhū nāma te sulabha vitthalarāj,
nivritti cheguja vitthal sahaja gainirāje maja sāngitale.

---

67. Ibid., XIII, 32.

"God, who is indivisible and self-existent, manifested every-where through chanting. Chanting very easily leads a seeker to perfection. My Guru, Gahiniraj, told me that my Vitthal, my Lord who is concealed, is my own Self." The Siddhas find chanting a nectarean *sadhana*.

The disciple loses himself in the teachings of the Guru. The Guru-disciple relationship is this: The Guru commands and the disciple obeys. Then the disciple becomes the Guru yet does not lose his discipleship. This is the perfect Guru-disciple relationship. It is based on the disciple's constant re-membrance of his identity with the Guru. Such a disciple ultimately becomes a great Guru. The Guru's position can-not be had cheaply.

The Search for Love

A person should forget his delusion and meditate on his own Self. There are only two ways to live: One is with con-stant conflict, and the other is with surrender. No victory can be won in life through conflict. Conflict only leads to anguish and suffering; no one has ever seen a person attain anything else from it. But when someone surrenders with under-standing and equanimity, his house, hands, and heart become full. His former feeling of emptiness and lack disap-pears, and his shortcomings are eliminated.

You hope to gain victory through outer love. You keep searching for it patiently, thinking it will bring you joy. But to lead your life with this wrong understanding is a sign of defeat. It is incorrect to say that the path of worldly life and the path to the bliss of liberation are different. You should understand both, because if you have only one kind of understanding you will be vanquished. You want love, but where are you looking for it? Think—have you missed your path?

Nasrudin was sitting on a bench in a garden, sound asleep and snoring, while his two companions talked about fishing. Their conversation soon became heated, and they began to fight.

One said, "Don't fish here. This is my place."

The other one said, "No, no, this is my territory. There are more fish here."

The first one snapped, "No, it's mine." They kept arguing in this way while Nasrudin continued to sleep.

In the meantime, a policeman arrived, saw the two men fighting, and woke up Nasrudin to ask him what was happening.

"O Mullah Sahib," he asked. "Why are these two peacocks fighting?"

The *mullah* replied, "O Policeman Sahib, please take both of them away so I can get some sleep. They are so smart that they're fighting about fishing here, where there's not even any water."

This is what happens to people: They try to fish for love where there is no water. Is this not what you do? Think about it honestly. Draw the map of your life and look at it in its entirety. What have you attained? Where is the love you have been seeking? Gain the proper understanding; give up your habit of complaining all the time. Learn to regard pain and pleasure as equal, and your complaints will come to an end. A Sufi saint, Bayaji, said, "How can one who cannot get out of hell go to heaven?" and "One who does not understand the darkness of night cannot understand the light of morning." Only he who has seen that the light of morning lies hidden behind the darkness of night can know and attain love.

A simple and natural love dwells just behind your complaints about the difficulties of worldly life. If you pursue meditation, knowledge, and equanimity, all your obstacles will disappear. If you rid yourself of mental conflict, then whether or not you go to a shrine, a temple, or another holy place, your prayer and worship will bear fruit, and love will begin to flow spontaneously wherever you may be. Desire will arise no more, and your search will come to an end. This is the path that leads to attainment. Empty your heart and purify it. Once love manifests within you, you will understand that you and everything else are perfect. You will see that perfection appears perfectly even in imperfection.

The Mirror of the Guru's Eyes

If through ignorance and wrong understanding you remain without a Guru, you betray yourself. Shri Guru loves you, whether directly or indirectly. No one can give you love as the Guru can. The love that you experience in your mundane life is petty and short-lived. A petty love has a short life span, and when this love departs, hatred arises. But nothing can equal the elixir of the Guru's love. In scriptural descriptions of the initiation process, there occurs the word *darshanat*, which means "through the Guru's look." There is a great mirror in the Guru's eyes, in which everything is reflected. The eyes are very active and reveal one's personality. The body can hinder one's self-expression because it is inert and gross, but the eyes are very subtle and offer no obstacle. Understand this completely: You can never deceive the Guru. Whether the Guru tells you so or not, your entire personality is revealed before his eyes. You are seen in every detail as in a clean mirror. You can be seen from any direction, for even when the Guru's eyes are closed he can perceive everything everywhere. You cannot hide yourself by looking away from him, and no matter where you may run the Guru's Shakti remains with you. This is why it is impossible to hide from the Guru. His Shakti will always follow you. Therefore, go to the Guru at least once, so that you can slow your pace.

When you are near the Guru, you may sometimes experience agitation. This is because of your ego, ignorance, weakness, and inability to recognize the Truth. When you agree to accept that Reality, when you establish a friendship with *so'ham* and learn to honor yourself completely, agitation dies and you experience utter peace within. But as long as you are unwilling to open yourself to the Truth, agitation will remain with you. This anxiety is caused by your own falsehood, your identification with the non-Self. A person who is untrue and who distrusts his own Self can neither sleep properly nor rest well. He can neither meditate nor love. As long as a person does not fully recognize the truth of his own inner being, he remains in constant turmoil. Lack of knowledge of the Self is hell. One's own ignorance is the architect of the city of hell; no one else creates it. To be in hell is simply to live in ignorance, while to be in heaven is to live in the ecstasy of the Self.

Jesus told his disciples, "Come to me and I will give you rest." Jesus himself was true and had attained perfect rest; he knew that there is an abode of perfect rest within. Falsehood is the kingdom of tension. Every evening many people who come for *darshan* tell me, "My mind is tense and restless." Husbands and wives complain that there is a storm of discord between them; they say, "Baba, do something." The Self is hidden from you because of your mental conflict and your distrust of your own inner being. What can you do? Give up your mental restlessness through the power of the Self. If you act without that power, your life is without stability. The only way to experience real peace is to give up your identification with the body and revel in the Self. When I tell people to do this, they reply, "That is very difficult." But it is not difficult. It is your everyday experience that if you have a conflict with one person, you find someone else; you eliminate the old conflict and for the time being put off thinking about any new conflict that may arise. In the same way, you can give up your identification with the body.

Throw away all attachment and aversion. Stop rejecting universal brotherhood. For a few moments, discard tension, restlessness, and jealousy, and quiet your mind. Turn within just for a while and make friends with the Self. Then watch how quickly you will be transformed. You will become simple and straightforward. Everyone will be yours, and you will belong to everyone. You will be able to do your work efficiently and with great freshness and ecstasy.

The teachings of the Guru are filled with virtue. Follow them, for they bring joy. In the beginning you may find the understanding that he teaches somewhat difficult, but later on that understanding will bring supreme bliss.

Do not be afraid. Fear has cut you off from the Truth. It has made you distrust the Guru and has taught you that you are ordinary. It is not easy to find a Guru, but if you succeed, open yourself to his compassion and try to follow the right path. Because the Guru is filled with compassion, if you absorb yourself in him compassion will also fill you. Immerse yourself in him with love and the feeling that he is your own. Tukaram Maharaj wrote:

deva mājhe mī devāche he chi mājhe satya vāche.

"God belongs to me and I belong to Him. I speak the Truth." You should learn to feel, "Shri Guru belongs to me and I belong to Shri Guru." This is the sublime relationship between the Guru and the disciple.

The Road to the Self

The goal of *sadhana* and religion is not discovered through idle chatter. It is very difficult to speak about that goal or about the knowledge that one has attained. There are no words for it; languages are man-made, while the ultimate state is total silence. One who tastes the goal remains mute; one who proclaims himself as God is only playing a role and revealing his lack of understanding of God. Trying to describe that inner state is, as Narada says in the *Bhakti Sutras, mūkā svādanavat*[68]—"like a mute person [trying to] describe taste." In the *Bhagavad Gita*, Lord Krishna said the same thing. Lao-Tzu spoke of this matter with truth and simplicity in many different ways, and Lord Buddha also described it very accurately from his own experience; he spoke eloquently about the real *dharma* and in this way benefited humankind. The only authentic teachings are those of a being who has genuine knowledge, who has come to understand That completely and has become serene. Such a being always points out the true path to others. Still, it is not enough to talk about the Truth. Such talk is only a supremely pure indication of the right direction to take.

In the *Bhagavad Gita*, the Lord exhorts us to become free of ego. We have become the playthings of ego. Not only do scholars, teachers, and those who talk about knowledge and meditation fall victim to ego; that subtle ego also makes them advisers. We never take the time to think about this, but the number of counselors in the world is amazing. Everyone is eager to become a guru and give advice; everyone is interested in healing. People are even ready to give out free advice, since the number of those who want it is so small. It is said that the thing which is most often given away is advice.

One day when Mullah Nasrudin had become very old, he went to a doctor. All his habits had been his comrades throughout his life. A person's habits never leave him in his old age; habits become the friends of one whose company they keep, and then one must have tremendous strength to discard them. The great being Bhartruhari expressed it well. *Yāvat svasthamidam kalevara-gruham:*[69] As long as the body is healthy, young, and strong, one can overcome bad habits. One should bear this in mind: If one is weak, what can one do?

---

68. *Narada Bhakti Sutras*, 52.
69. Bhartruhari, *Vairagya Shataka*.

Nasrudin was staggering, and his breath reeked of liquor. The doctor said, "Nasrudin Sahib, you are beyond treatment. For your own good, stop drinking liquor and smoking marijuana. Go home early at night and stop chasing girls."

Nasrudin stood up, thanked the doctor, took his stick, and started to leave.

The doctor cried, "Wait! Where is my payment?"

Nasrudin replied, "I would pay you if I were going to take your advice. As it is, there are people on every street corner who give it out free!"

Still, whenever there is someone giving advice, there are people willing to take it; some people will even listen to a blind man's advice. But a person should try to find out whether the one offering advice follows his own advice or simply gives it to others. Think about this and understand it: Why do you need to accept another's advice when everything that exists is within you?

A person who gives advice should have the experience with which to back it up; otherwise, how can he be an adviser? A person who lacks experience does not have the eye of knowledge; he has only a web of words, which is very dangerous. If one has not attained knowledge, if one's behavior does not befit a wise person, then one should not try to teach others. That kind of teaching is nothing but rubbish—the odds and ends of the world.

Faith is sublime. In the *Bhagavad Gita* the Lord says, *shraddhāvān labhate jnānam*[70]—"One who has faith attains knowledge." However, knowledge alone is not enough; along with it, experience is essential. Experience of the Truth has more value than knowledge, because contentment lies only in experience. In the same way, it is not enough to have trust in the Self; one must also have the experience. How can one have real trust without experience? This experience should be obtained from a Guru, for he alone can bestow it. A

---

70. *Bhagavad Gita,* IV, 39.

scholar threatens everyone with scriptures, but the Guru awakens people with knowledge.

There is a simple mystery behind the *sadhana* given by a Guru who is pure, well-behaved, vigorous, and true. Such a *sadhana* will lead you to perfection and Truth. Understand its secret. Keep walking on the path. Do not look behind you or very far ahead; otherwise, you will become frightened. If you keep walking, you will reach your destination. Then you will find that the Guru is with you and you are with him.

Let me tell you a simple fact. If you set aside your ego for a moment, you will realize that you, the traveler, are that which you are seeking. Everything is within you. The supreme inner stillness, the thought-free state, is your destination. It is God, the Self, Consciousness. It is the Guru as well as the disciple. It is the Guru-disciple relationship.

True Meditation

In the *Bhagavad Gita* it is said, *dhyānenātmani pashyanti*[71]— "Through meditation the Self is seen." Meditation is a subject for lengthy discussion. We meditate to attain our own Self, but in reality we attain that which we have already attained. To know this through right understanding is meditation. In fact, meditation is not something separate from our daily existence, but a part of it. Meditation is the means to a happy life.

Tukaram wrote, *tathasta te dhyāna*—"Meditation is total stillness." If one meditates deeply for one hour each day, the intoxication that results from it will last for the other twenty-three hours. But one's meditation has to be so deep that the waves of the mind become still.

---

71. Ibid., XIII, 24.

Someone asked a great being, "How should I meditate?" He replied, "Perform every action with total concentration. That is meditation." When you walk, you must do so with vigilance and complete concentration; otherwise, you will either miss the path or keep tripping as you go along. When you drive a car, you must be one-pointed, paying strict attention to the road and the highway signs; if you miss the turn-off you will miss the right road, and then you will be in trouble. In the same way, chanting inwardly, you should eat your food with total concentration, as though eating were everything. When you stand or sit, you should do so with complete absorption. All your activities should be carried out in this way. This is meditation. Whatever your work or service may be, you should do it without laziness and without caring about the time it takes to complete. Work done with great vigilance is also meditation.

The mind should not wander outside the present moment; rather it should stop within the boundaries of the moment and become completely still there. If, in the name of meditation, you merely sit somewhere with your eyes closed and allow your mind to wander all over town, you are simply wasting your time. True meditation is remembering the Self in the midst of all activities. As long as the mind continues to flow outward, your meditation will not be consummated even if you go to a temple, a mosque, or the Guru's house; even if you live in an ashram. If you remain unconscious in your home, in your shop, or in the market, how can you suddenly become conscious in a temple? A great being said that meditation really takes place only if it continues twenty-four hours a day. You should always maintain the inner recollection of meditation; then your meditation will be continuous.

Kashmir Shaivism teaches, *ita vā yasya samvittihi krīdāt-venākhilam jagat*[72]—"The entire world is the play of Universal

---

72. Vasugupta, *Spanda Karika*, II, 5.

Consciousness." If the inner stream of this awareness begins to flow, know that you are in the state of meditation. In this state, talking is meditation, eating is meditation, and going to the market is meditation. Let the mind merge into the awareness of equality. Once meditation happens in this way, joy will pour out of you.

Jnaneshwar describes meditation in this way: One fuels the furnace of self-inquiry by hearing about the Self, contemplating the Self, and thinking only of the Self. One burns up the impurities of the non-Self in the fire of knowledge and thus purifies the Self. In reality, of course, the Self is eternally pure. However, by burning the impurities and *karmas* created by the duality of the thirty-six *tattvas*,[73] one extracts the gold of the Self through the knowledge of the Truth. Shri Krishna told Arjuna that some seekers see the Self in the Self through knowledge of the Self. Others see the Self through the path of devotion, through the contemplation of Sankhya and Vedanta, through Siddha Yoga, or through karma yoga performed selflessly and with an attitude of service. (Service is a sublime form of meditation, knowledge, and yoga, and one should understand its mystery.) Lord Krishna said that in this way people attain God by different means and are saved from drowning in the ocean of worldliness.

The great seer Narada wrote, *labhyate'pi tatkrupayaiva*[74]— "This is attained through the grace of great beings." Through the grace of the Guru, one easily attains the state of meditation, which is filled with love and the welling up of great bliss. When Shri Guru sows the seed of *shaktipat* in the field of the heart, it sprouts into a plant, a tree, or a creeper and bears full fruit. The seed of the Guru's Shakti enters one very subtly and, by awakening one's inner Shakti, automatically gives rise to inner yoga. It does extensive work in one's body,

---

73. The principles of the different stages of the manifestation of the universe. See the Glossary for more details.
74. *Narada Bhakti Sutras*, 40.

reveals infinite miracles, and gives one a new life. *Shaktipat* is true life. It is rejuvenation. It is the alarm that awakens one who is dreaming in the sleep of worldly life. The *Katha Upanishad* says, *uttishthata jāgrata*[75]—"Arise and awake." For a long time you have been sleeping. Now awake! When Siddha Yoga, or the Guru's grace, awakens a person, he becomes happy, discards his illusory hopes, and opens his eyes to the day of knowledge. When a person awakens through the Guru's grace, he sees God. Then he becomes one with Him while still in this human form and is filled with joy.

The Delusion of Seeking

People earnestly go here and there in search of God, and that is very good, for if one is to lead one's life correctly one must find Him. However, some people become bored and give up their efforts. Moreover, just as some people consider a horse to be an elephant, there are those who have strange notions about God. Some consider Him to be a joke. Others even reach the point of saying, "We gave birth to God." The time will come when these people will proclaim, "I gave birth to my father," considering this to be a new, improved method, a new way of being clever, and a sign of the new age.

Looking outside yourself for God is merely foolishness. God exists in your understanding, which means that God is within you. You yourself are the inner thought-free state, *aham*, the pure "I"-consciousness, which is God. Hearing this, you may be amazed and wonder, "How can it be?" But that is your wrong understanding. The *Bhagavad Gita* says, *ātmaiva ripurātmanaha*[76]—"One becomes one's own enemy."

---

75. *Katha Upanishad*, I, 3,14.
76. *Bhagavad Gita*, VI, 5.

Through such wrong understanding, you create enmity toward your own Self.

If a person sets out thoughtlessly in search of God but does not find Him, why should this be surprising? New York cannot be found on the West Coast of the United States, because it is on the East Coast. You will never find God by searching outside, because He is inside you.

I will give you another illustration. One night a man took a lamp and determinedly set out in search of fire to dispel the darkness in his house. When the neighbors saw him, they laughed and said, "You're crazy! You have fire right in your hand. What is the use of looking somewhere else for it when you can light a fire with the lamp you're carrying?" The man instantly realized his mistake.

Such incidents often occur in our lives. For example, a person is wearing his glasses but forgets about them and asks, "Where are my glasses?" Looking through his glasses, he begins to search for them. If he were not already wearing glasses, how would he be able to see in order to look for them? Similarly, a clerk, a manager, a teacher, or a writer will often put his pencil behind his ear, forget where it is, and then look for it. When he discovers the pencil, he is relieved, yet he finds the pencil not because he was searching for it, but because he remembered where he had put it. In the same way, you should remember that your happiness, your bliss, and your God all dwell within you.

Once a group of villagers got together and decided to go looking for God. The next day, there was a ceremony in their honor. Of course, Nasrudin attended it. Three days later, an enormous crowd set out on the pilgrimage, and the villagers who remained gave them a big send-off. Suddenly, Mullah Nasrudin came riding at top speed through the market on his donkey. The villagers asked, "Nasrudin, where are you going?"

"Brothers, don't stop me now," he shouted. "When I come back, I'll tell you."

Nasrudin rode his donkey up to the crowd of pilgrims. He stopped, greeted them, and mounted his donkey again. The pilgrims asked, "Why are you in such a hurry?"

"I am thinking of going with you," Nasrudin replied, "so I am trying to find my donkey."

"Nasrudin, you are sitting on your donkey!" the pilgrims said. "Don't you understand? You're looking for your donkey even though you're sitting right on top of him!"

Nasrudin said, "In the same way, you're all looking for God while He is right within you! Why do you leave yourselves out when you go looking for Him?"

When Nasrudin returned to the market, the people there asked him, "Why were you in such a hurry?"

"I wanted to join the pilgrimage," he said, "so I was looking for my donkey, but the pilgrims told me that I was sitting right on top of him.

"Maybe I'm ignorant, but aren't you also fools? I couldn't find my donkey because I was looking for him off in the distance. But *you* could see him. You should have told me I was sitting right on top of him!"

The people in the market said, "You didn't give us a chance. We asked you where you were going, but you were in too great a hurry to tell us!"

This sort of incident has occurred in everyone's life, and since it is a matter of your own experience, you can easily understand how you can be looking for something that you already have. Although you live in Consciousness, you have forgotten it. Such forgetfulness is worldliness, while remembrance is spirituality; it is God. Just as fire cannot lose its heat, you cannot lose your Consciousness; just as water cannot lose its coolness, you cannot lose your state of *satchidananda*—absolute existence, consciousness, and bliss. Remember this, for it is the truth. Because you have forgotten it, you have forgotten everything—your worthiness, your Consciousness, your upliftment. Sometimes you have forgotten it to such an extent that you have been completely unable to recall it.

Mullah Nasrudin's landlord once told him, "Nasrudin, you borrowed money from me six months ago and still haven't shown any signs of returning it. Have you forgotten about it?"

Nasrudin replied, "Sir, give me a bit more time and I'll certainly forget it. When you keep reminding me every month, you don't give me a chance to forget it!"

Religious stories have many applications. They are priceless. In the scriptures ideas are explained at great length, but in a brief anecdote the same ideas can be explained in a few words. A story carves out an image in one's mind which helps one to remember the ideas it conveys. For this reason, the ancient sages would draw the complete map of a lengthy subject in a brief story. Such poet-saints as Kabir, Tulasidas, and Mira related long historical episodes in short poems and in this way sketched images in people's minds.

The Guru's Mantra

The mantra that one receives from the Guru has a mighty power. Through the mantra, meditation comes very easily. Mantra repetition always brings spiritual progress; this may take time, but do not worry. Repeating the mantra does not destroy the intellect, but strengthens it. As one repeats it, the intellect is purified and ultimately becomes the mantra itself. In the *Bhagavad Gita*, Shri Krishna makes clear the place of intellect in spirituality when he says, *dadāmi buddhiyogam tam yena māmupayānti te*[77]—"[To those who are ever-steadfast] I give the yoga of the intellect, through which they come to Me." By means of the mantra, the intellect becomes subtle, sharp, and rational, and one's understanding and way of thinking acquire new depth. The mantra turns the current of the intellect in a new direction.

---

77. Ibid., X, 10.

Ultimately, it takes it to *paravani*, the fourth and subtlest level of speech, from which the mantra arises. That is the goal of your search, the final stage of meditation, the place of recognition of the Truth. When you reach this place, the world will reveal its divine mystery before your eyes. You will see a pure, blissful, and enchanting sight, and then you will remember the Upanishadic mantra *īshā vāsyamidam sarvam*[78]—"It is God who pervades the form of the universe." When you become a true human being, you will become God. The movements of your thoughts will subside, and the doubts that lurk behind all thoughts will flee.

But remember that as long as you place your trust in the ego, the mantra cannot bear fruit and you can neither be purified nor perceive the Self. Cast off your ego. When it has been broken and blown to the winds, you will become truly open for the first time. As you open yourself, God's power will unfold and you will experience Him; your head will sway in ecstasy. How can the Truth have any value if the stream of bliss does not flow from it? Because the great beings understood this, they said, "Seek bliss." There is no point in wasting your life trying to discover the nature of the Truth. If you find bliss, you will also find the Truth; the Truth will present itself before you just as it is. Have this understanding: "I am the Truth; I am That." Practice the mantra *so'ham*. It will certainly give you that experience.

What Is Greater Than the Self?

The great sage Yajnavalkya told his wife, "Maitreyi, I no longer want to be a householder; I want to go beyond that way of life. I am going to leave and divide my wealth between you and my first wife Katyayani."

---

78. *Isha Upanishad*, 1.

"O lord," Maitreyi said, "if your wealth becomes mine, will I become immortal?"

Yajnavalkya replied, "Wealthy people have money, houses, gold, and silver and lead their lives accordingly. Your life will be like that, too. However, the hope of obtaining rest through wealth is simply a waking dream."

In the *Katha Upanishad*, it is said, *na vittena tarpaniyo manushyo*[79]—"A person is not satisfied by wealth alone."

Maitreyi asked Yajnavalkya, "If wealth will not make me immortal, why should I want it? You know the secret of immortality. Teach it to me."

"You are my beloved wife," Yajnavalkya said. "In addition, you are asking a question that is very dear to me. Come, and I will reveal this knowledge to you. But do not let what I say go in one ear and out the other. Pay complete attention to me.

"O Maitreyi, a wife loves her husband not for his sake, but for her own sake. A husband loves his wife not for her sake, but for his own sake. A father loves his son not for his son's sake, but for his own sake. One loves wealth not for the sake of wealth, but for one's own sake. One loves a priest not for the priest's sake, but for one's own sake. One loves a king not for the king's sake, but for one's own sake. One loves a deity not for the deity's sake, but for one's own sake. One loves all creatures not for their sake, but for one's own sake. Everything is dear for the sake of one's own Self. O Maitreyi, one should see and hear the Self; one should contemplate and meditate on it. When one does this and understands the Self, then everything is understood. Maitreyi, everything is attained through the Self."[80]

Our main difficulty in discovering the Self is that the mind does not want the supreme bliss of unity. Instead, it wants duality, and this duality is the source of all our problems.

---

79. *Katha Upanishad*, I, 1, 27.
80. *Brihadaranyaka Upanishad*.

Once Sheik Nasrudin was accused of theft, and the case was taken to court. The judge, who was very kind, said, "Nasrudin, it has been proved that you committed a theft. You have admitted your guilt, so now I will allow you to choose your own punishment."

Nasrudin replied, "You may give me any kind of punishment except that of being married to two women at the same time."

When the judge heard this, he was taken aback. "I don't understand," he said.

Nasrudin explained, "In the house where I was caught stealing, there were two wives, one living upstairs and the other downstairs. As I was leaving, I came upon the husband standing in the middle of the stairway. The wife who lived downstairs was pulling him by one hand, and the wife who lived upstairs was pulling him by the other. There was so much confusion and trouble that I was not able to escape. The husband and his wives were at an impasse, and I, poor thief, was trapped upstairs. The suffering I saw that night was sufficient punishment. Now I am ready to accept gladly whatever other punishment you care to give me."

All life's sufferings are the result of the mental torment that arises from the sense of duality. When one is experiencing conflict, one's entire life becomes painful, and one does not know a moment's peace. The mind suffers when it has even one desire; when it has two or three desires, it suffers infinitely. Yet as Vedanta says, everything is one; there are not two. Anyone who sees two suffers, so give up the idea that there are two and then discard the one that is left. When both are cast off, that which remains is eternal; it is the Truth which no one can erase. That Truth is you. It is Consciousness. It is also called *atmaram*, the Self. It is your true nature. You should have the desire to know that Self because as long as you fail to do so, as long as you have not seen the fundamental and sublime Truth of your life, you will remain deluded no matter what you do.

Remember this as long as the sun and moon exist: No one but your own Self is at the heart of your joy. As Yajnavalkya told Maitreyi, one loves one's husband or wife not for his or her sake but for one's own; in fact, a devotee loves God not for the sake of God, but for his own sake, for the sake of his own Self. *Ātmādadhikam kimasti tattvam*—"What principle is greater than the Self?" Your own Self is the center of everything. Day in and day out, everyone in the world spins in all four directions trying to find the answer to the question "Who am I?"

Swami Ram Tirth was a great being who was good-natured and had faith in the Self. He asked himself, "Who am I? Around whom do the sun, moon, stars, shadows, day, and night revolve? Who am I? In whom do morning and evening appear? In whom do the stars arise? Who am I? Unless I know this, I will be utterly incomplete. As long as I do not discover who I am, then no matter what I do I will be like a man walking in the dark, thinking that something lies ahead."

Such blind movement can never take us to our destination. Where do we look for our goal? The goal lies within us, yet we always search for it outside. A husband looks for it in his wife and a wife looks for it in her husband, both mistakenly thinking it must be in the other. Sometimes the goal appears to be in a particular place outside, but ultimately the Truth lies within us. That Truth—the illuminator of all our inner senses, the revealer and the witness of our waking and dream states, the one who understands our understanding, and the knower behind the knower—is our own Self. It is the Self of Rama, of Krishna, and of the entire world. Because of the Self, all actions, religions, sects, incarnations, sages, yogis, and seers exist. Our only obstacle to finding the Self is the fact that we are looking for it outside ourselves; to think that the goal is outside is a sure sign that we have been deceived. When a person breaks through this deception, then for the first time in his life rays of light shimmer in all directions—rays of knowledge, bliss, and an ecstasy that is oblivious to all else.

Therefore, Yajnavalkya told Maitreyi, "O Maitreyi, whether through meditation or knowledge, you should realize that the Self exists in your own heart." The heart is the hub of all existence. If we look for that center outside, we will continue to wander for infinite lifetimes. Just think! So many eons have passed. Since the beginning of creation we have been roaming about, but we have never found that center outside, nor will we ever find it there. The truth is that if the Self could be found outside, we would have done so long ago. Today, not only do people travel all over the world, but they have gone to the moon and investigated Venus. Yet they have not found the Self, for the Self lies hidden within the one who is seeking. It is not something we can hold in our hand, for it is intangible. It is not something we can see, because it is the seer. It is impossible to touch the Self, because it is the Self that touches. Moreover, when we turn within during meditation, we realize that the Self cannot be found by seeking because it is that which seeks. Knowledge of the Self is withheld from one who tries to know it. However, the Upanishads say that when one knows it, everything is known, and this is absolutely true.

One should meditate with respect, and see, hear, and contemplate the Self. The Self is the sole basis not only of one's own life, but of the entire world. Everything rests on this foundation, which in Kashmir Shaivism is known as *samvitti*, Universal Consciousness. Only the Self deserves to be contemplated with such respect and vigilance. This is why the eyes of the great beings slowly close to the world when light and bliss begin to manifest within them. One who sees the Self sees everything. It makes little difference whether one sits in meditation with one's eyes closed or open. One's attention must be turned within for the work to be done. Nonetheless, one should know that it is already done; the Self is already attained.

The Inner Intoxication

There is a mantra that describes a being who is established in the Self: *antarlakshyo bahirdrushtihi nimisho' nnimisha-varjita-gatihi*—"[one] whose eyes are unblinking and whose gaze, though appearing to look outside, is fixed within." In this way, although our eyes may appear to look outward, our gaze should be directed within. We should also turn our hearing inward. Meditating yogis slowly direct their outer hearing toward the divine inner music and listen for a long time to the divine inner sounds, or *nada*. The Upanishads refer to this *nada* as *om*. *Om* is not merely a mantra to be repeated; it is the sublime and indestructible sound of the Self which continuously reverberates within us. It is the divine music of our true inner existence arising spontaneously without two objects being struck together. It has been resounding since the beginning of time and is the eternal Truth. The entire universe exists within this sound. Because it exists, all the activities of the world take place. It makes the sun rise and set and the wind blow. The creation, maintenance, and dissolution of the universe occur within this vibration, which in Kashmir Shaivism is called *spanda*, the original throb. One who wishes to know it must hide his eyes from outer forms and colors. He must shield his tongue from outer tastes, and his nose from outer fragrances. He must free his hands from outer contacts. Only then will he experience that divine vibration.

Jnaneshwar Maharaj wrote, *indriyāsi choruni heye tayāsi pāve*—"One tastes and attains this elixir by stealing it from the senses." When the senses become free from all outer contacts, for the first time in one's life one experiences the inner sensation of joy that lies at the core of one's being. When one sees and hears one's Self, one touches that inner love. When one tastes one's own Self, one experiences *sat-chidananda*. Whoever has tasted this sublime elixir has tasted the mystery of life and the essence of the entire world.

The divine sage Narada said, *yadjnātva mātto bhavati stabdho bhavati ātmārāmo bhavati*[81]—"Knowing this, the devotee becomes intoxicated and still, reveling in the Self." By attaining and experiencing the nectar of the Self, which is supreme love, one becomes ecstatic. One who is completely established in the Self becomes utterly quiet and serene; he becomes the Self. When the love of God, the ambrosia of the Self, is revealed, one finally attains the Truth and begins to dance like a madman. The intoxication that arises from the love of the divine Self is overwhelming. I often say, "Why do you use marijuana, opium, and cocaine? If you want real intoxication, drink the elixir of the Self. That will take you higher and higher; you will never come down from it."

When a flowing river merges into the ocean, it becomes the ocean and so takes on the ocean's delight. The ocean of the Self is complete in itself. Intoxicated with love, it billows ceaselessly with its own joy. A person who is immersed in the Self becomes drunk with love. Sometimes he dances out of sheer joy. Sometimes he is lost in a state of overwhelming bliss. At other times, he is engrossed in discussing the Self. Narada said, *amruta svarūpāchcha*[82]—"The love of the inner Self is nectarean by nature." That inner love is not far from us; since its source lies within us it is not, and cannot be, concealed. We ourselves have obscured it. Our blindness makes us think that it is hidden, but it is manifest within us.

Wandering in the Kingdom of Thoughts

We are unable to experience the Self because of the thoughts in the mind. The mind can never stop thinking; thinking is its life. Day after day, it continually dwells on external

---

81. *Narada Bhakti Sutras*, 6.
82. Ibid., 3.

objects—on a shop or a market, on a friend or an enemy, on wealth.

A great Siddha named Jonaid was staying in a certain town at the home of a Moslem priest. Jonaid was God's servant and a perfect Guru, but he never went to mosques. The priest had made many attempts to persuade him to go, but Jonaid always laughed and let the matter drop. One day a special religious festival was held, during which thousands of people gathered to do *namaj*, the Moslem prayers. On this auspicious occasion, the priest was so insistent that Jonaid come to the mosque that he could no longer avoid the issue. "Alright," he said. "Since all places are the same, it makes no difference to me whether I am here or there." Jonaid's outlook was correct. He was always immersed in the love of God and thus spent every moment in *namaj*.

"If it will make you happy, then I will go to the mosque," Jonaid told the priest. "But remember, I am going for your sake. I've never seen you go to the mosque, so I don't know where it is. You will have to come with me."

The priest was taken aback. "Of course I will come. I go to the mosque five times a day."

Jonaid replied, "There is a difference between going to the mosque to worship and going because it is your occupation. You go to a mosque the way a shopkeeper goes to his shop. You insist that I come with you, so I will submit to your demand. I've never provoked you before, but today you have trapped yourself.

"I will go with you," Jonaid continued, "but you must agree to do *namaj* with me. Only then will I give in to you; otherwise, I will cause trouble."

The priest could not understand Jonaid. He thought, "Of course I'll do *namaj*. I do it five times a day; I'm a priest!"

When Jonaid and the priest reached the mosque, everyone began to do *namaj*. However, instead of kneeling, Jonaid remained standing. Suddenly he began to bellow like a buffalo. Everyone in the mosque opened his eyes in amazement, for Jonaid was a highly respected renunciant who had attained Siddhahood. The priest became nervous and upset, regretting that he had brought Jonaid. But Jonaid went on bellowing louder and louder, as if a buffalo were speaking from within him.

When he could bear it no more, the priest cried, "Jonaid, that's enough! You have spoiled everyone's *namaj*. What kind of game is this? I never knew that you lacked understanding!"

How can people who keep track of the time during prayers, recitation, and worship understand the state of an ecstatic being who is absorbed in love for God? Someone once asked Tukaram Maharaj, the crest jewel of saints, "Maharaj, how does a fish sleep in water?" Anyone who asks a great saint so impudent a question has no intelligence. Does he not show a lack of understanding? To ask such a question is neither *satsang*, chanting, a meditation technique, nor a means of crossing over the world. Tulasidas said that such a person always has bad thoughts and a quarrelsome mind and lives in hell. Nonetheless, Tukaram's reply was very beautiful: "If you want to know how a fish sleeps in water, you will have to be born as a fish."

In the same way, an ordinary person who lacks understanding cannot know the mystery of a Siddha's state. It takes very subtle vision to understand it, and not everyone can have that vision. In the *Bhagavad Gita* Lord Krishna says, *bahūnām janmanāmante jnānavānmam prapadyate*[83]—"A man of knowledge attains Me after many lifetimes." Only an enlightened being, only one who has eliminated his impurities and faults by performing virtuous actions and pleasing God, only one who has done *sadhana* and conducted himself very well for many lifetimes can understand God and other enlightened beings.

The priest again told Jonaid, "That's enough! What is this game?"

---

83. *Bhagavad Gita*, VII, 9.

The great Jonaid replied, "Remember, you insisted that I come with you. I warned you that I would do *namaj* only if you did it and that otherwise I would cause trouble. But if you can only think about buffaloes, what can I do? I am simply following your lead."

When the priest heard this, he was shocked. It was true that he had been absorbed in thinking about buffaloes. For a long time he had wanted to buy a buffalo for its milk, but he had not had enough money. Since today was an important festival of prayer, he expected to receive a large amount of money. During *namaj* he had been calculating how much he would receive and thinking about the buffalo he would buy the next day. He had been picturing in his mind the many different buffaloes he had seen in the market, trying to select the right one.

Jonaid asked, "Tell me the truth. What were you thinking about during *namaj*?"

"Forgive me," said the priest. "I made a mistake. I shouldn't have brought you here. It is true that I was thinking about buffaloes while outwardly doing *namaj*. What an extraordinary man you are! You really are an omniscient, ecstatic being. Every time I pictured the face of a buffalo, you bellowed."

One should not pursue meditation in the way that the priest performed his *namaj*. Instead, one should become completely absorbed in prayer, meditation, and contemplation and lose oneself in them. Narada said:

yatprāpya na kinchit vānchati na shochati na,
dveshti na ramate notsāhi bhavati.[84]

"After attaining love, a person has no desire for anything else." A being who has found the inner love neither suffers nor becomes excited over trivial matters. He neither hates nor becomes attached to anything. Why should he become

---

84. *Narada Bhakti Sutras*, 5.

trapped in delusive dramas when he holds the source of the world, the center of bliss, in his hand? Why should he take interest in the wrong path? Why should he be attracted by a market where buffaloes and sheep are sold? Why should he criticize any religion, sect, or person? A *mahatma* who does such things is false, a mere imitation. People should be extremely careful and use their intelligence and power of reasoning when they approach a spiritual being.

Some gurus give their disciples teachings about sex. But why would one need lessons on that subject? Someone once asked me to give him some understanding about sex. I said, "This is very surprising. Aren't you married?"

"I used to be, and I have a child," he replied.

"You ignorant fellow!" I said. "After creating a child, why do you need to ask me about sex? Even the animals in the jungle procreate without asking questions." Be ashamed of gurus who give teachings about these things. What can one attain from such gurus?

An incident similar to the Jonaid episode is told of Guru Nanakdev. (One often finds certain incidents occurring in the life of more than one great being, for these beings share the same behavior and customs, as well as the same correct outlook.) Guru Nanak used to say, "Hindus and Moslems are one. Temples and mosques are the same." Once a Moslem landowner heard these words and asked Nanak, "If that is true, why do you always go to a temple and not to a mosque? You say that temples and mosques are the same, so prove it by coming to the mosque with me today."

"Since you insist," said Nanakdev, "I will come, but only if you will also come."

The Moslem replied, "Of course I will come. Let's go. All the Moslems in the village have gathered."

While they were walking down the road, Nanak said, "You must also do *namaj*; otherwise, I will not do it."

"You don't have to tell me to do *namaj*," the man said. "I've been doing it for so long—why would today be any different?"

When they entered the mosque, Nanakdev remained standing. He would not do *namaj*, nor would he bow down. The landowner was upset. He did his *namaj* quickly and then began to rail at Nanakdev. "What you say is all nonsense! It's not true that Hindus and Moslems are the same! By refusing to do *namaj* with me, you are supporting the idea of religious differences."

"Were you really doing *namaj*?" Nanak asked. "You kept opening your eyes and looking at me. So instead of doing *namaj*, I also watched you. Does your *namaj* consist of watching me or watching God? The truth is that you were thinking about me. You didn't think about God even for a moment."

When you practice contemplation, meditation, and chanting, are you really doing these things or are you dwelling inwardly on mundane matters and thus pursuing the yoga of the world? Is your journey of meditation and knowledge only taking you toward the world? Ponder this with great subtlety. Turn your mind within. Seek your own inner Self, the true friend of the mind. You must use the friend of the mind for the sake of the mind; you must make the Self the mind's companion.

The sage Yajnavalkya said, "O Maitreyi, the Self should be fully seen, contemplated, and meditated upon." Anything else is useless. Wandering continuously in the kingdom of thoughts is not meditation; it is merely playacting in the name of knowledge and meditation. Only when one becomes centered in the original core of one's being is one truly meditating.

All your life, energy flows out through your senses. Turn the senses within, if only a little, so that you can hear, know, and contemplate the inner divinity. When That is known, everything else is known.

Pursuing the Master

The emphasis in spirituality is on attaining complete knowledge of the One, whereas science emphasizes the study of many different subjects. Science is concerned with multiplicity, whereas spirituality is concerned with oneness. Science involves the analysis of one branch of knowledge after another, while spirituality involves contemplation only of the One and, in that way, gives rise to wisdom.

What did Lord Shankaracharya, Lord Buddha, Nanakdev, Kabir, and Jnaneshwar not know? What did they not understand? They mapped out the entire world from top to bottom, in all its aspects. They fully understood time and its effects and extracted a single essence from everything they knew. But if we were to ask them questions about our mundane lives and activities, they would not be interested. If we were to try to draw them into long scientific discussions, they would consider us ignorant. If we were to ask them why hydrogen and oxygen combine to produce water, they would not have the slightest desire to know the answer. Truly, there would be no point in asking these great beings about worldly matters. Having come to understand that which contains all knowledge, they would find no reason to take interest in lesser forms of knowledge.

> *yenāshrutam shrutam bhavati amatam matam,*
> *bhavati avijñātam vijñātam bhavati.*[85]

"By knowing [That], the unheard is heard, the unknown is known, and that which is beyond understanding is understood."

People make assumptions about the nature of the Truth but are far from understanding it. It is difficult to know That; in fact, most people who make the attempt ultimately give up and set out in a different direction. However, when one understands That, everything one was previously un-

---

85. *Chandogya Upanishad,* VI, I, 3.

able to understand becomes understandable. That has manifested in many aspects, all so different from one another that they do not appear to be connected. But when one knows That, the desire for all other kinds of knowledge is fulfilled. When That is known, whatever was not known becomes known. When That is heard, whatever was not heard becomes heard. These great beings—Lord Shankaracharya, Lord Buddha, Nanakdev, Kabir, and Jnaneshwar —knew and assimilated That completely. They understood the Master and clung to Him and thus came to know everything. *Yasya sarvam idam vasho*—"[The Lord is He] under whose control all this is." When these beings assimilated that which controls everything, they became absorbed in total peace and attained satisfaction.

But while they pursued the Master, we pursue servants. There are many servants, and even if we happen to find them, we can win nothing from them. Ultimately, our hands remain empty. We remain imperfect, lacking steadiness and possessing only indecision and doubts.

Once a sovereign was preparing to return home after a successful military campaign. Before he left, he sent a message to his twenty wives saying, "I have won a great victory. Let me know everything you want; I will return with presents for all of you." Each wife wrote him a letter listing the objects she desired. One wanted jewelry set with diamonds. Another wanted jewelry set with rubies. Another wanted gold, and still another wanted perfume from abroad. One wanted this, and another wanted that. Each had her own preference. This is how a person lives. Lacking knowledge of the Truth, he chooses things according to his own interests without understanding whether they are good or bad for him. All his life, his interests continually change according to his whims, which indicates that he never really finds what he wants. Yet the *Bhagavad Gita* says, *yadjñātvā amrutamashnute*[86]—"Knowing [That], one attains nectar."

---

86. *Bhagavad Gita*, XIII, 12.

By experiencing the Self, one is filled with the highest bliss. Once one attains that which is supremely interesting, one finally becomes satisfied.

One of the king's wives sent him a blank sheet of paper along with a letter. In the letter she wrote, "I want nothing except my beloved husband. The palace is empty and dark without you. Come back as soon as you can."

A person lives in his own desires and hopes, but who knows what will happen in the next moment? That is why the great beings try to awaken us; it is the task of Gurus to awaken those who are sleeping in delusion.

jāg re nar jāg pyāre abto gāphil jāg re,
māyā kā jāl bichāyā hai, lambe isase bhag re,
kāma krodha ahamkār trushnā, sanga inaki tyāg re,
dekha le ranga rūpa terā, guru-charan-anurāgare.

Here the great being Brahmananda warns, "O dear one, awake! O ignorant one, awake now! The net of *maya* has been cast. Flee from it. Give up the company of desire, anger, lust, and ego. See your own true Self. Love the Guru's feet." The Gurus tell us again and again, "Awake! Perceive your own Self. That which you are seeing now is a magic show, a carnival of *maya.*"

The king filled a boat with all the objects that his queens had requested and set out. It would have been much better if he could have traveled by jumbo jet, but those were different times. During the voyage a violent storm arose, and the boat sank with all its goods. Only the king himself managed to escape and, with great difficulty, to reach the shore. The wives who had asked for worldly objects got nothing. The one who had asked for the king himself got him as well as the kingdom.

Our voyage across the ocean of the world is difficult. With her voice full of yearning, Mirabai begged the Lord:

nāv kināre lagāvo prabhuji,
nadiyā gahari nāv purāni, āp hi pār lagāvo.

"Take my boat to the shore, O Lord! Deep is the river; old is the boat. Take it to the shore." When the time finally comes, one's boat will sink along with one's world. Only the Master will be saved. If one does not beg for His grace, one will die in poverty. If one calls out for Him, one will find Him within oneself. Then it will not matter whether the boat sinks, because nothing will have the power to take away one's freedom and identity with the Master. One will become the sovereign of the free, divine, and perfect kingdom of the Self. That kingdom contains ever-new vitality and the ecstasy of life; it is a world full of bliss.

In the *Vishnu Samhita* it is said, *yasya vijñāna-mātrena ānanda-lakshano mokshaha prāpyate,*[87] which means that one attains the bliss of liberation through knowledge of That. Then everything is attained; there is nothing else to be done. *Yadvidvān na bibeti kutashchana*—"A person who knows That is afraid of no one."

This is the true mystery of the Supreme Self. One does not have to go anywhere to search for it, because it exists within one's own heart. It is God's nature to be fully satisfied within Himself; in Him there is neither dissatisfaction nor desire. Therefore, Narada said, *yallabdhvā trupto bhavati*[88]—"Attaining That, one becomes contented." One experiences complete satisfaction; there is no more thirst. Tukaram Maharaj expressed it correctly: *thān bhūkha harapale tujā pāhatā vitthala*—"O Vitthale, when I saw You, both hunger and thirst were eliminated." When one comes to know God, there is no more asking, no more begging, no more praying. On the day when one becomes God, one's prayers cease.

Narada said, *tanmayāha*[89]—"A devotee becomes immersed in God," and *tasmin tajjane bhedābhavataha*[90]—"The difference

---

87. *Vishnu Samhita,* 2.
88. *Narada Bhakti Sutras,* 4.
89. Ibid., 70.
90. Ibid., 41.

between God and the devotee vanishes." Tukaram Maharaj said that in this state, duality becomes unity. When all one's prayers cease, when all one's begging is completely eliminated, one finds that which is worthy of being attained right within oneself.

The Inner Silence

As long as the mind is not completely quiet and thought-free, one cannot know the Self. Jnaneshwar wrote, *mana mure muga jo ure, kāhere tu tyālā sevecha nā, dīsate pari kalecha nā*—"Why do you not worship that which remains after the mind is eliminated? You can perceive it, but you cannot understand it." Through intense concentration, one should experience the inner silence of the thought-free state. Then the inner veil will be lifted, and the door that has been closed for so long will be opened. When light penetrates darkness, suddenly there is light everywhere.

As long as the mind is not completely still, you have nothing more than the hope of joy. When you are speaking to others, you can at least choose to stop talking, but you have no control over your inner chatter. Even when you want to stop your mind, you cannot do so because it is not under your control.

What is the real meaning of madness? It means having no self-control. A person in this state is entirely dependent. He cannot change what is happening now or what will happen in the future, nor can he cause something to happen. He has lost his self-mastery; his life is ruled by his senses and his mind. Having fallen under the control of his ego, he gossips endlessly and speaks pretentiously: "I'm so rich; I'm so virtuous; I'm such a great writer; I'm so wise." Such a person is the slave of his mind; his mind and his desires have conquered him. From this standpoint, we are all the friends of madness. There may be some difference in degree. Some people are crazier than others; some hold themselves together with a bit of discipline. But everyone is the friend of madness.

Once Lord Buddha was asked, "Are you God, or a deity, or a special incarnation?"

Lord Buddha replied, "I am none of those things. I am the one whom you know at the moment you awaken from sleep, when you are free of thoughts."

What profound understanding! A being with this kind of knowledge has awakened from the madness of the sleep of ignorance. Knowing no disparity or conflict, he is the image of joy—a complete human being. Such a person is called a great being, a knower of the Self. We must all awaken in this way.

To converse with others we have to use language, but to speak within ourselves we need no outer language. When we wish to speak with love, the language we use is silence.

The scriptures say, *gurostu maunam vyākhyānam shishyāstu chinna-samshayāha*—"The Guru lectures in silence, and the disciple's doubts are removed." The Guru's silent speech destroys all the disciple's doubts. The glory of silence is limitless; nothing is so powerful. One who has observed the ancient truth of silence has nothing more to attain. In silence one realizes that one is the perfect Self, the embodiment of Truth and Consciousness. Pushpadanta said, *atītaha panthānam tava cha mahimā vāngmanasayor:*[91] The glory of the king of the Self is so sublime and extraordinary, so profound and mysterious, that it transcends the mind and speech. The mind and speech are forced to turn away from it, because there, where one's inner Truth lies, only silence is speech.

Silence is the highest religion and a symbol of the eternal Truth. Everything else is subject to destruction. Old weapons are destroyed and new ones are fashioned. Old scriptures

---

91. *Shiva Mahimna Stotram,* 2.

are destroyed and new ones come into being. Scientists are always disproving old theories and discovering new ones. People die. But the Truth is unfailing. It is old in the old and new in the new. It is the truth within the Supreme Truth; it is the you in you, the ultimate state of the perfect inner "I"-consciousness, the blissful thought-free state. It does not need the scriptures and has nothing to do with them. Even if the scriptures were destroyed the Truth would be unaffected, because the Truth produced the scriptures; the scriptures did not produce the Truth. The Truth is beginningless, infinite, and perfect.

Words are the means by which we know objects. But to know God the supreme silence of the thought-free state is essential. To attain that thought-free state is the purpose of *sadhana.* One who tries to journey there by giving lectures will miss the path, for articulated speech is gross, and the gross can never grasp the subtle. Birth and death both take place in silence. Silence is true life. Talking to others can be useful, but it will never reveal one's true nature, for that can be known only when one completely lets go of duality. There is no point in merely forgetting words; one must forget duality. To give up words means to go within, and that means losing all remembrance of one's conventional identity. Once words go, language also goes, and one should understand that one has then learned everything. Memory is useful for mundane activities and for giving lectures, but only forgetfulness will help one attain the Self.

The Need for the Guru

The Guru's help is essential to one who wants knowledge of the Self. Without the wisdom of the Guru, the notion of one's individuality will never be rooted out. Without the Guru's grace, one cannot be uplifted, and without the Guru's knowledge, the darkness of one's ignorance can never be destroyed. All individuals are bound by the noose of time, but one who keeps the Guru's company will not feel the blows of death. Kabir Sahib said that without the Guru, birth and death will never be annihilated. Without the Guru, life is full of darkness. For many lifetimes we have been trapped in worldliness; only the Guru can release us. We should contemplate this and understand it. The subtle path to the Self is most easily attained through the Guru. Kabir said that the Guru makes one perfect; he unites the individual soul with Shiva. Therefore, one should keep the company of the Guru and remain respectfully at his feet. When one has his *darshan* and listens to his words, delusion flees and cheerfulness, joy, and compassion arise. Gurudev is like the philosophers' stone; he makes his disciples just like himself. This is the true Guru-disciple relationship.

Darkness is nothing new in this world; it is familiar and ancient. Equally ancient is our search for light. The more we are steeped in darkness, the less we are able to find light. But at the same time, it is as impossible for one who is in darkness not to yearn for light as it is for one who has been hungry for a long time not to desire food. Just as a hungry person naturally wants food and one who is thirsty searches for water, the desire to find light in the primordial darkness is ageless. But although you have set out on your journey in search of light, you have not yet found even one ray. You have searched for a long time, wandering from temple to temple, from mosque to mosque, from mountain to mountain, from ashram to ashram, from course to course. You have sown the seed of seeking, but you have not yet reaped the harvest of discovery. This is the truth.

A person who walks in darkness does not know light; how can he look for light when he has never seen it? In which direction will he travel? If he tries to discover a path by himself, he will simply go around in circles, walking for a long time but never reaching his goal, attaining only a mountain of fatigue. That is why if you want to reach your spiritual destination, it is important to ask someone about the path. You are wrong to think that you will accomplish anything on your own. Unless you leave your individuality behind, you will not be able to find the way. If you continue to search independently, you will find only darkness; you will think your own thoughts and remain locked in your own experience. Therefore, it is absolutely certain that you need a wise guide. Seek the help of one who knows the light, who has experienced it, in whose life the current of its nectar flows, and who has become supremely satisfied by attaining it. The significance of the Guru is that he has found everything you are seeking; that which you want has become the Guru's wealth. The difference between you and the Guru is that you are the seed and the Guru is the full-grown tree; you are the beginning, and he is the end. Inherently, the only difference between you is that one step.

The world is an extraordinary drama. The *Shiva Sutras* say, *nartaka ātmā*[92]—"The Self is an actor." The world is God's theater, God's play, and the sport God has created for His own pleasure. A person who understands this understands everything. For him there is no room for duality or enmity and no reason for hatred. Any form of duality is merely ignorance, the gift of the great *maya* and the friend of the god of death.

There are many proud, egotistical, and arrogant people in the world who say, "I am very wise; I am superior to others." Such people are playthings of *maya*. They are not true human beings. They may ask you, "What is your problem? Who is the God you are seeking? What is this meditation? If such a thing exists, why do I not experience it? Prayer and worship are nonsense. Liberation is a dream. Why do you sit in *siddhasana?* Why do you waste your time sitting cross-legged in the name of God? For whom do you sit with your eyes

---

92. *Shiva Sutras*, III, 9.

closed? No one is going to come to you. Why do you go to temples, mosques, and other places of prayer? No one is there. This is all a trap of the theologians. You read the scriptures, but they are only a scheme of the shrewd and a play of the clever. Do not get entangled in these involvements. There is no problem. Do not worry about contentment. Why do you go to a Guru? We are intelligent people. Live your life as we do. Eat well, drink well, consider your senses guests, and spend your time satisfying them. Live in this world making merry, eating, and earning money in whatever way you can. Have fun. Get high in clubs. If you get sick, go to a doctor and take medicine. If he cannot solve your problems, go to a psychologist, and if he cannot help you, take drugs." Many people say such things.

There is something that you should remember: A person who becomes aware of his own ignorance is drawn to the Guru's feet, but the pride of knowledge gleaned from dry books leads one to look for scriptures rather than for a Guru. Although the scriptures emphasize surrender, vows, and discipline, they are lifeless, so one does not really have to surrender to them; one can interpret them in any way one likes. But one cannot interpret the Guru. You may change the scriptures, but the Guru will certainly change you. He will begin by awakening you, by telling you that you have forgotten your own Self. Lacking knowledge of your Self, you are deep in the sleep of ignorance. The Guru will open your eyes to your darkness, ignorance, and forgetfulness. Only after knowing darkness is it possible to find light. Only one who falls can get up. Unless a seeker knows what it is to fall down, it is difficult for him to rise. After the Guru has made you aware of your condition, he will give you the vision of your own Self.

The Destroyer of Fantasies

Kabir wrote, *gurudeva vinā jīvaki kalpanā na mitai*—"Without the Guru, fantasies cannot be rooted out." Fantasy is the world of *maya*, the dream of one who is sleeping, and no matter how beautiful and enchanting it may be, it is still a dream and therefore unreal. An ignorant person lives in a false world of fantasies, considering someone to be his friend when there is actually no one to befriend him, imagining that someone belongs to him when no one is really his. Although he is standing close to death, he believes that he possesses eternal life. Although wealth is dangerous, he regards it as everything and yearns to obtain it. Although the body lasts no more than a few years, he becomes completely immersed in it, thinking, "I am going to live in this body forever." The currents of his thoughts are no more than gusts of wind, yet he becomes so engrossed in them that he believes, "All this is everlasting." He pays respect to the almighty ego and surrenders his entire life to it. Under the influence of this false ego, he is ready to kill and be killed, considering the victory of ego to be his success. This fantasy is simply ignorance.

In the same way, a seeker gets caught in the fantasy that he has come to understand the Truth. A scripture says, *anubhūtim vinā mūdhaha vruthā brahmani modate*—"Without experience, a fool takes delight in Brahman in vain." An ignorant person who has not experienced the Truth pretends that he knows Brahman when actually he does not, and then he performs his play for others.

This sort of knowledge is *pratibimbita-phala-svādavat*—"like tasting the reflection of a fruit." On the bank of a river was a mango tree whose fruit was reflected in the water. Once an unmindful person came by and tried to mentally taste the reflection of the mangoes. In the same way, illusory knowledge is meaningless, a mere mental process. It is fantasy to consider anything one's own.

The home of true knowledge is *satchidananda*; understanding the Truth means knowing and experiencing it as it is. You do not need great courage to see the Truth, because you are already That. The Truth is never displeased with you; it is always pleased. The Truth does not have to approve of your desires, because it always approves of you. It is not necessary for the Truth to fulfill your dreams; instead, it is important for it to shatter them.

Without the Guru, it is not possible for a person to understand the Truth, any more than it is possible for one who has given up *sadhanas* and spiritual practices to find That. Without the Guru, it is impossible to stop the eyes from looking outward, to stop the mind from casting its net outside, or to overcome and transcend the mind. Now, you keep chasing the dreams of your desires, trying to extinguish their flames, but instead of using the water of understanding you pour on the gasoline of desire. When you behave like this, how can the fire ever be extinguished? This is why Kabir said that without the Guru, a person's fantasies cannot be eliminated. You can change their form, type, and structure, but they will remain alive; you should not cherish any hope that they will be rooted out. You may think that you can do everything through your own cleverness. But if you rely on the endlessly expanding world, the most you can ever do is give up thinking about worldly matters and start thinking about liberation. This is useless, and you will attain little from it. First you will put forth effort, and then you will have the pride of illusory freedom; that will be your attainment.

Your fantasies can be eliminated only if you keep the company and receive the love, compassion, and kindness of one in whom the Truth is manifest. Ponder this and understand it. The heart of such a being is a temple in which God always dwells. Such a Guru takes you gradually, one step at a time, toward the Truth. Slowly, he releases you from your fantasies.

Once a great seeker named Nagalinga went to live with his Guru. At first the Guru talked to him sweetly and joyfully about the state of steady wisdom, liberation, the formlessness of God, Siddhahood, and other sublime matters. In this way, he created a dreamlike illusion in him.

Out of his desire to attain the Self, Nagalinga began to do rigorous *sadhana*. As a result of being in the Guru's company, he began, after a few years of practice, to experience meditation and to understand how to attain the Self. One day Nagalinga felt that if he took one more leap, he would attain Siddhahood. He went to his Guru and, touching his feet, said, "I want to take one more leap forward. I need a slight push from you, and then I will attain Siddhahood."

Very seriously and with great patience the Guru said, "What Siddhahood? What liberation? What *Brahma nirvana*? All this is just useless gossip."

Nagalinga became stiff with fear. "Gurudev," he cried, "what are you saying? I am practicing *sadhana* with great hope and faith."

The Guru replied, "We get children to go to school happily by giving them sweets. We do not give them sweets for the sake of giving them sweets, but so that they will go to school. When they start taking interest in school, we give them fewer sweets, and one day we stop giving them sweets altogether. It is the same with your desire to attain Siddhahood. Up to a certain point, fantasies were useful, but now you have to give them up. There is nothing to attain. You do not have to attain the One who is eternal and all-pervasive, who exists equally in all, who neither decreases nor increases, and who is always pure, because you have already attained Him. There is only one thing to do; you simply have to know Him. What is there to attain? He is always with you. Now, know Him."

At first Nagalinga was terrified. Every hair of his body stood on end, and he began to sweat. It is easy to renounce the world, but it is not so easy to renounce Siddhahood. The Guru continued, "Siddhahood is a pair of golden handcuffs. Give them up. Become simple and straightforward."

In this way, you must simply give up all your infinitely

varied and fanciful dreams. Let them go without a backward glance, just as a snake sheds its skin and never looks back wondering, "Where did I leave it?" When your visa expires and you leave the land of fantasies, the abode of liberation is right before you. You immediately realize the Truth.

Liberation and bliss do not conform to your desires, nor is true freedom a product of your dreams. Liberation resembles nothing you have ever imagined. You may try to contemplate and discuss it, but you will never succeed because it does not easily fit within the framework of your thinking.

> na tatra sūryo bhāti na chandra-tārakam
> nemā vidyuto bhānti kuto'yamagnihi,
> tameva bhāntam anubhāti sarvam
> tasya bhāsā sarvam idam vibhāti.[93]

"When the brilliance of even the sun, moon, stars, and lightning does not reach there, what can you say about fire? Everything is illumined and revealed by the light of That." The Guru, who resides in that place which no one can reach, will certainly reveal its light to you.

Therefore, before you set out on a pilgrimage to the Infinite, reflect upon your undertaking with great care. If you go alone, your journey will be confined to the realm of the mind. If you want to go beyond the mind, you will need a companion who has himself transcended the mind and can therefore take you by the hand and lead you on the journey. A small child needs a wise person to give him self-confidence and a helping hand, someone to kindle faith in his heart so that he can eventually stand up and walk straight on the path. Similarly, a seeker of Truth needs a strong hand and a firm support. Kabir wrote, samaj vichar le man mānhi rāha bārīk gurudevse pāīye: Think this over and understand it. The path is very narrow and precarious; it is so subtle that you need the Guru's help to discern it. Jesus also said, "Straight is the

---

93. *Katha Upanishad*, II, 2-5.

way and narrow is the path." Its subtlety is such that it is
beyond your experience and understanding. When this is
the case, how can you walk on it? You cannot find the path by
clever thinking; thoughts are not sufficiently subtle. As long
as you do not give up your mental cleverness, as long as your
thought-waves do not subside, you will neither recognize
nor experience the bliss of That. This is why Kabir said that
one needs the Guru's help in order to find the way.

When the kingdom of fantasies collapses, only the Guru
remains as the support of all. In one of his poems, Sunderdas
wrote, "The Guru has revealed the perfect Brahman, who
alone is all-pervasive. To whom can you be attached? Whom
can you hate? Whatever exists is That. The root of everything
pervades everything. All the thoughts and doubts of the
mind have been obliterated. Through the contemplation of
That, the Guru has firmly established me in the Truth. He has
washed away all my filth and made me pure. When I meditate on my Guru, my heart is filled with ecstasy."[94]

The Experience Beyond Words

Many people in the world think about God, but one does
not attain God merely by thinking about Him. Just as in the
sleep state there is no waking and in the waking state there is
no sleep, similarly, God cannot be found in thoughts. Thinking only leads to more thinking.

Many people complain to me, "Although I have been
meditating, reading, and taking different courses for a long
time, I still do not experience anything. If I feel any love, it
vanishes immediately and the same old negativities arise
again." I ask them, "On what do you meditate? If you were
to contemplate God while sitting for meditation, you would

---

94. *Sundervilas.*

certainly be purified. Instead, you think and contemplate without any understanding and therefore get nowhere. Understand this and be patient."

Whatever you have read about God in the scriptures is merely an indication of Him. By thinking about the scriptures over and over again, all that you have gained is the desire to attain God. Words are created by God, so how can He be known through them? *Nāpi pramāna-gocharaha*—"He cannot be perceived through scriptural proofs." Moreover, *tarkāpratishthānāt:*[95] Logical reasoning is of no use. God is not words; He is an extraordinary inner experience. The scriptures belong to Him, but He cannot be confined to them. Words can point the way to God, but He is far beyond them. He cannot be understood through the mind, the intellect, or the subconscious mind, yet a true seeker attains Him within himself through the path and the wisdom of the Guru.

God is the support of the world and has become the world; He pervades everything in it. He is the son and the daughter, the mother and the father; he is the entire family, including all the relatives. Heaven and hell emanate from Him. Everything—horses, grains, crops—belongs to Him, for He is everything. When a person casts off ego and the awareness of duality, he discovers that Shiva is not different from him. When one attains complete understanding of Him, one's awareness of the world merges into Him. The *Shiva Sutras* say, *sthithi-layau*[96]—"The maintenance and reabsorption [of the world] take place within God." Although *maya* does not actually exist, God is its foundation. He is One.

sarvānana-shiro-grīvaha sarva-bhūta-guhāshayaha,
sarva-vyāpī sa bhagavān tasmāt sarva-gataha shivaha.[97]

---

95. *Brahma Sutras*, II, 1, 11.
96. *Shiva Sutras*, III, 31.
97. *Shvetashvatara Upanishad*, III, 11.

"He who is in the faces, heads and necks of all, who dwells in the cave [of the heart] of all beings, and who is all-pervading is the Lord and therefore the omnipresent Shiva." In reality, it is God alone who assumes these various forms. He manifests many strange fantasies within Himself; it is He who makes the actress *maya* play her role. (*Nartaka ātmā*[98]—"The Self is an actor.") This creation is a play for His own delight.

In the *Bhagavad Gita* the Lord says, *samo'ham sarva-bhūteshu*[99]—"I exist equally in all." In this way, God's law is the same for everyone. It is flawless and impartial.

Think about this carefully: Are there different heavens and hells for each caste? Is there one for poor people, another one for middle-class people, and a first-class one for wealthy people? Are there special heavens and hells for Hindus, for Tibetans, for Jews, for Sufis, and for Christians? Of course not. How can there be different ways of managing things in heaven? The idea of caste exists in people's minds, and there are as many castes as there are ideas. But heaven and hell are the same for everyone. In the military everyone wears the same uniform, and in a court of law everyone is equal. Living is the same for everyone, as are sleep and death. God's law is only one. No caste can interfere with it, for God is supremely free.

As God is impartial, He is also generous. No giver in this world can equal God. A charitable person may give wealth, clothes, and a certain amount of help, but God is so munificent that He gives Himself. One who looks for Him becomes Him even while seeking Him. As Tukaram Maharaj said, *devāpavayāsi gelā tethe devācha hoūni thelā* — "I went to see God, and I myself became God."

God is *satchidananda*, the undifferentiated One without a second. He is the Supreme Truth, which is infinite and the

---

98. *Shiva Sutras*, III, 9.
99. *Bhagavad Gita*, II, 29.

life of the entire universe. One who does not know God does not know anything. But one who pursues Him through the mantra *hamsa-so'ham* becomes Him and is blessed. Such a person should indeed be called a great being. Once one knows God, one's old understanding is no more. Supreme bliss and joy lie only in knowledge of the Self. Ignorance of the Self is pain.

God is self-inspired love. Narada said, *prakāshate kvāpī pātre*[100]—"This love manifests spontaneously in a worthy person [with a pure heart]."

> *guna rahitam kāmanā-rahitam pratikshana-vardhamānam,*
> *avichchhinnam sūkshmataram anubhavarūpam.*[101]

In this aphorism, Narada explains that divine love does not depend on the *gunas*—it is beyond them. Having no desires, it seeks nothing in return. It is perfect and ever-increasing, it does not wax and wane, and it is free of any sense of duality. Because it is subtler than the subtlest, it cannot be described, but can only be experienced. This pure love expands from day to day. When one is deeply absorbed in thought, one is merely thinking, but at the very instant when one becomes free of thoughts, one experiences the pulsation of that inner love. Once one experiences it, it never departs.

This experience is attained through the Guru. As Kabir wrote, *sadguru mile samshaya sakala mitāi hridaya me rām lakai*—"I found the Sadguru, who removed all my doubts and revealed Ram in my heart." We should fully understand what it is that we are to attain from the Guru. By being with the Guru, we are not supposed merely to study the scriptures or just to go on thinking; we are supposed to attain inner meditation. The true meaning of meditation is becoming immersed in the thought-free state. This state is love; it is the Truth. We experience it when we are fully awake, when

---

100. *Narada Bhakti Sutras*, 53.
101. Ibid., 54.

all the clouds in our inner sky have dissolved, when there are no more thoughts and images to suppress and our inner space is completely empty, when the light of experience shines and the divine sun of knowledge blazes forth. We have to meditate on this state. It is the ultimate meditation, the true meditation, which can only be experienced, never spoken about. It culminates in natural *samadhi*.

The great king Alexander wanted to conquer India. Because ruling so small a country as Greece was not enough for him, he wanted India as well; a desire can be so great that even the three worlds are insignificant in comparison. Before Alexander left, he went to his guru Aristotle for his blessings. "I am going to invade India and conquer it," he said. "What gift should I bring you from there?"

"O king," Aristotle replied, "if you find a Guru who can extinguish the fire of our desires, bring him back with you so that enmity and violence can be removed and the rarest of all things, God's love, can be attained."

Alexander did not bring back a Guru; in fact, he never reached India. The invasion of India was merely a dream of his mind. However, Aristotle's words were true. It is through the Guru that the love of God is attained.

The Inner Transformation

Remember that as long as your clogged mind has not been cleaned out, as long as your vessel has not been emptied and washed, you will not be able to fill it with God's nectar, nor will you be able to digest that nectar. It is important that your vessel be empty and completely purified in the fire of meditation and knowledge.

I repeat that you can find the narrow path only with the help of a Guru; it is too subtle for an ordinary teacher to show you. An ordinary teacher can give you a limited kind of knowledge and teach you different meditative techniques, but only a Guru can give you inner meditation. There are many who can give you knowledge no matter what your condition may be. You can acquire a certain type of knowledge in a university or college; for that you need not stay in an ashram or in the Guru's house. That kind of knowledge is very cheap and can be found in any market or library. But remember one thing—the cheaper it is, the more useless it is. The fruit of cheap knowledge is insignificant. True meditation, however, is the best of all *sadhanas*. The *Bhagavad Gita* says, *dhyānenātmani pashyanti*, [102] which means that one can attain the Self through meditation. Meditation is a great technique.

Some people kindle the fire of discrimination between the Self and the non-Self. They spread the pure gold of meditation over the alloy of Self and non-Self. Through the fire of discrimination, they eliminate the dross of the thirty-six kinds of duality and bring out the gold of the Absolute Principle. By perceiving the knowledge of the Self, they see the principle of the Absolute as their own Self. This is the highest meditation.

It is difficult to attain the true state of meditation; the fact is that you reach that state only when you are completely prepared to erase yourself. Meditation first obliterates you; it kills you. But do not be afraid—meditation is not a murderer or a butcher or a violent assailant. The words of a saint will help you to understand this:

safā se milā jaba safā ho gayā main,
khudī mita gayi khud khudā ho gayā main.

"When I realized the Pure, I became pure. My ego was no more. I myself became God." When the saint discovered oneness, he merged into everything. When his ego was

---

102. *Bhagavad Gita,* XIII, 24.

annihilated, he himself became God. This is very mysterious. To die while still living is to become deathless and
immortal. Many people fear death, but in this sort of death
the individual soul becomes Shiva. It is not a literal death:
Meditation simply erases one's small self and thus makes
one God while one is still alive.

I read a verse in the Urdu language, *mitā do apne hastīko
agar tum kuccha martabā chāhte ho*, which says that if you
want to become great, you must first obliterate your existence. If you hold onto it, what will you be able to attain in
meditation? You will only retain your ordinary understanding, which is useless. A great being said, *ke dān khāk me
milkar gule guljār hotā*: A seed is sown in the earth and
completely disappears, yet it is not destroyed. It seems to be
dead but, in truth, it flourishes. In the earth, its individuality is transformed and it grows into an enormous tree full of
joy, love, and beauty. That tree has innumerable seeds
within itself, and thus by losing itself the seed becomes
immortal. However, if it preserves itself, it is annihilated.

Another great being said, *vo khudī ko mitāvo na tab tak khudā
nahi miltā*: As long as you have not destroyed your ego, God
is far away. Erase yourself; then you will find real meditation.
The source of true meditation is the Guru. I once read a poem
which explained that the Guru is death: When you go to him,
you have to die. It is not that the Guru is Yamaraja, the god of
death, who will actually kill you. The Guru bestows indestructible life. Nonetheless, when you approach him, your
false ego will certainly die and your false existence will be
annihilated. Sunderdas said that when the philosophers'
stone comes in contact with iron, it kills it. But it does this
only to give the iron new life by transforming it into gold. A
sandalwood tree is very fragrant and cooling; many people
use its oil. Moreover, it has the virtue of spreading its fragrance and coolness to all the trees that surround it. Sunderdas said that in a similar way, a Sadguru transforms a true
disciple. Then he attains true understanding, and his essen-

tial nature, which is perfect and full of joy, manifests. But this can happen only when the kingdom of fantasies is eradicated.

The Giver of True Knowledge

The current of love of *satchidananda* flows through the Guru. Without the Guru, inner knowledge cannot be revealed. Without the power of the Guru's grace, meditation cannot take place. Discipline does not automatically come into a person's life; it is through the Guru's grace that one acquires the virtues of good conduct and spontaneous contentment. Without the Guru, the thirst to attain God does not arise. The *Bhagavad Gita* says, *buddhi-grāhyam atindriyam*[103]—"That which is beyond the senses can be perceived through the intellect." But an intellect that is dull, that has been made impure by the filth of the world, does not reflect light. An illumined intellect can be attained only through the Guru. Unless the delusion of worldliness is destroyed, doubts never cease to arise and, again, only the Guru can shatter one's delusion. Just as one cannot buy anything without money, there is no true path without the Guru.

"I say this openly," wrote Sunderdas, "and this is the doctrine of the Vedas and the scriptures." Sunderdas was a great Siddha, and so was his Guru, Shri Dadu Dinadayal. Because of his knowledge of the Self and his awareness of equality, Dadu had neither enemy nor friend. To him everyone was equal. His attachment to the body had been completely transformed. The Self alone was everything to him, and he reveled only in the Self. He had no other involvements, activities, or outside enterprises. He did not

---

103. Ibid., VI, 21.

perform healings or give psychic readings; such things never happened around him. He lived uninterruptedly in the ocean of supreme bliss. Although supernatural powers stood at his door, he never raised his eyes to look at them. Sunderdas said, "Everyone listens to him. How can one adequately praise such a Guru? I offer my salutations to him."

In India there is a saying: "Drink water only after straining it, and accept a Guru only after coming to know him very well." A true Guru is not attached to anyone, nor does he harbor any feelings of enmity. He does not criticize others or discuss their faults. He is not violent and does not hurt anyone even by mistake. He shuns such chatter as, "I am great. I know everything. Call me God." He does not indulge in the give-and-take of business. He is partial to no one and does not secretly perform bad actions with anyone. He does not accumulate followers and tempt them to walk on the wrong path. He takes no interest in idle gossip; his sole delight lies in the contemplation of the Absolute. This is the state of a true Guru. Sunderdas said that such a Guru is the god of gods. He alone can be called the Guru and no one else. From him one attains meditation easily and simply.

Kabir wrote, *guru janam janam ke atak kholī*—"The Guru has freed you from being stuck for many lifetimes." The word *atak*, "to be stuck," is very amusing and likable. There is a wonderful mystery behind it that is well worth understanding. When one plays a record, the phonograph needle sometimes becomes stuck and moves in the same groove over and over again, as if it were doing *japa*. Just as it moves in the same groove without going either backward or forward, one can also become stuck in one's *sadhana*. Eon after eon, the "needle" moves in the groove of birth and death, pain and pleasure. But if someone lifts it and moves it over, the cycle comes to an end.

There is another way of becoming stuck. One day when

Kabir was young and wandering in search of God, he saw an old woman grinding grain into flour by the roadside. As he watched the flour fall from the grinding wheel, he began to weep. A great being named Nipat Niranjan, who had been observing all of this, went to Kabir and asked, "O child, why are you crying?"

Kabir answered, "All the grain that is put under the grinding stone is being ground. Not a single grain is saved. In the same way, the entire world is being ground in the huge grinding stone of time. I am crying out of fear. How can we escape from the grinding stone?"

Nipat Niranjan laughed and brought Kabir closer to the grinding stone. He told the woman to lift the upper stone. Then he pointed to the stick that connected the upper stone to the lower stone. "Look, Kabir," Nipat said. "The grain that is stuck at the base of the stick is not ground. It remains perfectly intact. If you want to be saved from the grinding stone of time, go to Kashi. A great being called Ramananda lives there. Stick to him. Then the grinding will not affect you, and you will be saved."

Guru janam janam ke atak kholī—"The Guru has freed you from being stuck for many lifetimes." If you stick to the Guru, he removes you from the groove of birth and death. One who sticks to him does not wander. There is a saying: *sab ghar bhatke gurunāth ghar atke*—"One wanders from house to house but becomes stuck [that is, steady] in the Guru's house."

Kabir wrote, *gurudev puran milai jīva aur shiva tab ek totai*—"Once you find a perfect Guru, you no longer perceive any difference between the individual soul and Shiva, between the Self and God." This was the teaching of the great Kabir. Shankaracharya also proclaimed, *jivo brahmaiva nāparaha*—"The individual soul and the Absolute are not different." The sign of a perfect Guru is that he does not see the slightest difference between you and himself, or between you and God. He will give you and God equal weight on a scale. Mira said, "I weighed Him on the scale, putting myself on one side and Him on the other." To give equal weight to God and the individual soul is the sign of a Guru.

The Delusion of Unworthiness

There are many prominent teachers in the world who praise God while continually criticizing others and their worldly life. Those teachers have neither known nor attained the Truth; they have acquired only book knowledge. They serve as a wall that separates you from God and create distance between you by saying that He is far away. They insult you, telling you that you are a vile sinner and giving you the impression that there is sin and wretchedness in the pure Self. As a result, you see yourself in the light of these impressions and live accordingly. A true Guru, on the other hand, breaks your old habits of faultfinding, of seeing sin, and of hating yourself. He roots out the negative seeds that you have sown as well as your feelings of guilt. He makes you rise above your imagination and discover the Truth. He explains to you, *tat tvam asi*—"Thou art That"—and thus makes you realize that God is you, that there is not the slightest difference between you and God. Such a Guru will take you straight to your God.

You will never hear the Guru criticize you. Instead, when you are in his company, you will experience your own divinity. You will never be found guilty in the Guru's eyes. You will find in them only the praise of your hidden inner God.

Kabir wrote, *sab ghat lāl bharā hai sūni sej na koī*: Every heart is filled with God; no heart is empty. The Sadguru's work is to make you understand this. That Sadguru is pure, compassionate, and righteous; he has not fallen from the true path. He knows and has followed his Guru's command.

Your liking for self-criticism is very strange. The assumption that one is unworthy does not suit a human being. Yet it is almost funny how much interest you take in that assumption and how respectfully you accept it. The *Bhagavad Gita* says, *tulya-nindā-stutir mauni*: [104] A great being who is a guide to the Truth remains unmoved by praise or blame. But do you belong to that category? Absolutely not! In fact, it is very likely that you do not know in which direction the Truth lies. It is amazing how much you like to criticize yourself. Not only do you relish the word "sinner," but you delight in other foul terms as well. Why do you like to put yourself down? It is because since childhood you have been hearing this kind of self-criticism in your society and from the people with whom you associate, and you have picked up the habit. The result is that you do not believe that you can be God. You do not trust that God is concealed within you. You think, "I am a thief; I am dishonest;" your conscience reminds you of your actions, and you keep mulling them over in your mind. Since you are so accustomed to belittling yourself, whenever you are criticized by a spiritual teacher you nod your head in agreement and sometimes even reply, "Yes, it is true."

Because you view yourself in this way, a network of detractors has existed for a long time. It seems that the more these people criticize you, the more you love them. In their lectures, these so-called great teachers shower abuse on their audience, saying, "You are thieves and phonies. You are all filled with anger and greed." Nonetheless, the members of the audience are very pleased; they applaud and nod their heads. When will this kind of misunderstanding leave you?

You may find the Guru's words difficult to accept. They do not conform to your experience because you think of yourself in terms of your old ways of being. When the Guru tells you, "Friend, God is within you; in fact, you are God," you

---

104. Ibid., XII, 19.

remember the deceitful actions you have performed and think, "How can I be God when I have done all these things?" Faith cannot grow in you because you know your own falsehood too well. But your knowledge of yourself is the knowledge of a dream; it is not true understanding. You do not know your real, essential nature.

Once the great Swami Ram Tirth was traveling by night on a ship. The sky and the ocean were dark blue, and the moon and stars shone. Filled with the awareness of the Self of the universe, this great being was joyfully contemplating the presence of God in his surroundings. While he was singing and swaying in ecstasy, a man sleeping by his side was having a nightmare about a tiger with three large horns. When the tiger attacked him, the man woke up with a start, sweating with fear. He turned to the swami and cried out, "Swamiji! Where did the tiger go? He attacked me ferociously!"

"What tiger?" the swami asked. "This is a passenger ship. Where could a tiger possibly come from?"

"I just had a dream about it!" the man cried.

"How could I see your dream-tiger in my waking state?" the swami said. "The tiger was only a dream. It wasn't real."

All the Gurus—Kabir, Nanak, Tulasi, Tukaram, Jnaneshwar, Ekanath, and so on—said that everything one does, whether good or bad, is a product of a prolonged dream. Your true existence is beyond the boundary of your dreams. Wake up! Then you will be free from your imaginary dream.

The Mystery of Satsang

Nanakdev said, *bāhar bhītar eka hi jāno yaha guru jnāna batāī*—"The Guru gave me the knowledge that the inside and the outside are one." Keep the company of the Guru. The term *satsang* is very powerful and important to understand. It originated in India to describe the company of holy people and saints. Having *satsang* means being with the Guru or being close to him, but more than this it means becoming one with the Self of the Guru. To merge with the Guru is to become perfect within one's own Self. For this it is enough to have the awareness of the oneness of the Self, the sense of the Self, the feeling of *pūrno'ham*—"I am perfect."

Scientists make use of catalysts in their work. A catalyst is a substance that causes other substances to change without itself changing. The Guru acts as a catalyst. He does not have to do anything; to experience his effect, you merely have to be in his presence. Bathe in the radiance of the Guru's Self. Come to him and be immersed in his experience of oneness. For a moment, become his companion and journey to the realm where he roams. Bathe for a while in the holy river of his love and understand that when you do this, everything is accomplished. You are perfect. You are the Truth. Kabir wrote, *karo satsang gurudeva se*—"Keep the company of the Guru." God becomes one with a person who has drunk the nectar of *satsang*, who has great love for *satsang*, and who through *satsang* has attained the kingdom of the supreme state of liberation.

There may be many great *sadhanas* for attaining God, but *satsang* is the most sublime. It bears fruit instantly; in fact, all *sadhanas* bear fruit because of it. Through *satsang* one's desires are fulfilled; one learns to meditate ceaselessly on the Supreme Self and then does not have to do any other *sadhana*. Knowers of the Truth, great yogis, and enlightened beings with equal vision have *satsang* and become serene. Such beings have become divorced from pride. As a result of *satsang*, they have washed away all their sins and, by hearing the great statements made during *satsang*, have forever banished their doubts. Keep the company of those saints. When your faith in *satsang* increases, liberation will come looking for you.

Being with the Guru is a great art. You must be very

intelligent, and you must possess great courage and contentment. Although laziness, desires, and lack of faith may besiege you, you should never ask for anything. The question of asking should not even arise, for if you ask for something it will take you far away from the Guru. Stay with him, requesting nothing. Do not wonder when you will attain the Truth. Pray, meditate, and wait patiently with love. Learn to forget yourself in meditation. *Satsang* is very mysterious. If you simply stay in the Guru's company with great care, the right time will eventually come, and then you will attain perfection. Everything has its own season for ripening, and yours will also arrive. When the Guru's glance of grace and compassion falls on you, you will become ripe.

The Guru is a burning flame. That flame lacks nothing, nor is it diminished when it lights an unlit wick; even if thousands of flames are lit from it, it is not affected. When you want to light a candle, you bring together a flame and the unlit wick. As you bring them closer and closer, a leap occurs, and the wick is lit. This takes only a fraction of a second. The moment for you to become something will come sooner or later and then there need only be a leap. Therefore, have *satsang* at the Guru's feet. *Tasmād brahmaivāchārya-svarūpenāvatishthate*—"It is Brahman who exists in the form of the Guru."

The only way to attain *satsang* is to surrender yourself. You must leave the future of your *sadhana* to the Guru. Give up the desire to become something, because if you enclose yourself in your own desire, your sense of individuality will prevent the Guru's Shakti from entering you. Let the Shakti penetrate you. Become simple, or you will remain bound. To come to the Guru you must be worthy, but if you have a pure heart and inner faith your delusion will flee at the mere sight of him. Look at him well. When your eyes meet his, you will have the vision of your own inner Self.

A true Guru considers wealth to be dust, and the world of duality a stomachache. He considers the company of false people to be the death of one's wisdom. For him, wanting to become important and obtain respect is committing a sin against the truth of universal equality. He regards both good and bad fortune as nothing more than the mistakes of his past. Although people show him respect, he accepts it reluctantly, considering it a curse. He regards greatness and praise as insults. He considers heaven to be as hot as fire, and Brahmaloka[105] an obstacle to supreme bliss. For him fame is a blemish, and supernatural powers are thieves of knowledge. He harbors no desire for anything because he has become free of desire. Sunderdas said, "I offer my salutations to one who has this kind of understanding, and I have *satsang* with him."

You can detect a perfect Guru if you look at him with perfect vision. When you see him, you experience an inner throb and you understand that you have seen your own Self. Truly, the Guru functions as a mirror in which you see your own reflection. In the Guru, you see and attain your own Self.

This brings to mind one of Ram Tirth's stories. A rich man had constructed a palace of mirrors that was open to anyone who wished to go in and look at himself. Once a genuinely enlightened person entered and looked around. When he saw his own reflections he thought, "It is I who exists in infinite forms," and became very happy contemplating the all-pervasiveness of his Consciousness. Later, a dog came in. When he approached the mirrors, he saw countless other dogs staring at him. He became terrified and began to bark. When he looked up, thousands of dogs were barking at him. When he looked down, thousands of dogs were barking at him. In his terror at the sight of them, he barked and barked until at last he dropped dead.

Like the man in the palace of mirrors, an enlightened being sees only equality. In order to teach in the worldly realm, a Guru also has to perceive duality existing within

---

105. The world of Brahma, the highest of all the planes of heavenly existence described in the Indian scriptures.

the fundamental unity. But he himself has become free of duality; if he has not, you will not attain anything from him. The Guru can be a perfect mirror only if he has erased himself. He must be one who has become completely free of thoughts, who has transcended the void, and who is established in the state of the Witness. The Guru is a lake whose waves have disappeared. As you come closer and closer to him, you will not find him; you will find only the light of your own Self. As you begin to understand the Guru as a mirror, he will show you your Self. The divine inner sound as well as love, understanding, peace, and discrimination will burst forth within you. This is the explosion of so'ham, the experience of the Infinite, the knowledge of the Truth. When this explosion took place in Mansur Mastana, he cried, anal-haq—"I am God!" When it occurred in Shankaracharya, he said, aham brahmāsmi—"I am the Absolute," and told everyone, "You are that which exists forever. You are Consciousness; you are God." This is the primordial explosion. The world was created by it, is maintained by it, merges into it, and then manifests again. The old merges in it and is reborn as the new. This divine explosion or vibration, which is the power of sound, is known as spanda, the cosmic throb, and has been resounding since time immemorial. When you perceive it, your delusion will flee, and joy, love, and compassion will arise in your heart.

When you see your own Self in the mirror of the Guru, all your needs are satisfied and you understand that you are supremely free. Your desire to perceive the Self is fulfilled, and you feel boundless love for the mirror. Love for the Guru will never leave you, for he is your own reflection, your Self, your eyes, and your vital force. How can your love for him disappear? When you see your own Self, supreme devotion to the Guru arises and a new age begins for you.

A person who has seen the Self is transformed. All his bad feelings dissolve like the morning dew that vanishes when the sun rises. His violence also leaves him, just as old skin falls away from a snake or as darkness abandons a house the moment a lamp is lit. When a person attains the Self, then virtues, discipline, and all the divine qualities come looking for him and take up residence within him.

A saint said, "If a person receives the Guru's grace, what can time do to him?" Jnaneshwar wrote, "After one sees the Lord of the universe, the knot of one's individuality is removed." The moment a person sees the Self, both death and the fear of death are annihilated for him. He has brought about the death of death itself. Death remains alive only in the understanding of one who does not know the Self. When a person understands who he is, the apparent duality between God and himself dies. The death of duality is the attainment of immortality; a person who has attained his own Self knows that his essential nature is deathless. He begins to sing and dance, exclaiming, "I have found God within myself!" Darkness also dies, and he experiences light and nothing but light everywhere.

Remember that your ego is death, whereas the knowledge of the Self regenerates you. When you revel in the Self, your delusion departs, and then there is no more birth for you, no more returning to the world. You become immortal in this very body and in this very world, experiencing the immortal realm in all your actions and associations. However, in order for this to occur, the heart must be fully ripe. Ripe, juicy fruit falls from a tree by itself, and similarly a mature mind easily merges into the Self.

The Natural State

All *sadhanas* as well as *samadhi* and the awareness of equality should take place naturally. It is neither natural nor correct to make an effort to meditate and get into *samadhi*. A state of *samadhi* that is forced is not particularly remarkable;

in fact, it is a betrayal of true *samadhi*, a deception that one chooses along with one's practice. This kind of *samadhi* occurs only when one practices a technique, whereas true *samadhi* and equality-awareness are not dependent on anything. A person carries out all his daily activities effortlessly and with love—it is natural for him to sleep, natural for him to wake up, natural for him to sit, and natural for him to eat. To be immersed in one's own Self as effortlessly as one is immersed in one's ordinary actions is the state of natural *samadhi*.

Everyone has his own sense of himself. A doctor knows, "I am a doctor." A professor knows, "I am a professor." A designer knows, "I am a designer." A *sannyasi* knows, "I am a *sannyasi*." These people never lose their natural understanding of themselves even when they are playing, singing, or engaged in any other activity. In the same way, once one recognizes one's true nature through the Guru's grace, that recognition remains with one at all times and in all actions. Kabir wrote:

sādho sahaja samādhi bhali,
guru pratāpa jo din se jāgi,
din din adhika chali.

"Natural *samadhi* is superior and sublime. Once it is awakened by the Guru's grace, it continues to grow day by day." On the other hand, when *samadhi* is attained through one's efforts and rigorous practices, it remains difficult for one to transcend the mind, because those efforts and practices belong to the realm of the mind. That which one attains through the mind does not take one beyond the mind. That which one attains through one's own efforts will not be any greater than oneself. In the *Kena Upanishad* it is said:

yan manasā na manute yenāhurmano matam,
tad eva brahma tvam viddhi nedam yad idam upāsate. [106]

---

106. *Kena Upanishad*, I, 6.

"That which is not thought by the mind but by which
. . . the mind thinks—know that That truly is Brahman
and not what people here adore."

*yach chakshushā na pashyati yena chakshūmshi pashyati,
tad eva brahma tvam viddhi nedam yad idam upāsate.* [107]

"That which is not seen by the eyes but by which the eyes
see—know that That truly is Brahman and not what people here adore."

*na tatra chakshur gachchhati na vāg gachchhati no manaha,
na vidmo na vijānīmo yathitad anushishyāt.* [108]

"There the eye goes not, speech goes not, nor the mind; we
know not, nor understand how to teach about That." That is
Brahman.

It is difficult to attain Him through exertion; if a person
could attain God through his own seeking, God would be
inferior to him. One cannot attain God without erasing oneself. As Kabir wrote, one can realize Him effortlessly through
the Guru's grace and compassion. But to seek God without
grace is to lose Him.

It is important to understand how the state of *samadhi* can
be reached in a natural manner. The great being Ranganath
Maharaj said, *sahajo me sahaj samane ki aisī yukti sabhī ko nahi
ānekī:* Not everyone has the ability to attain that natural state
spontaneously. Only great beings like the Guru possess that
skill and can pass it on to others. The fact is that God is not
much concerned with the different kinds of spiritual activities, with one's effort, or with rigorous practices. Whoever
has attained Him has said that he realized Him through the
Guru's grace.

Thousands of people used to come to see my Gurudev
Shri Nityananda. They would sit very quietly and in silence
while he played in the ecstasy of his own inner love. He

---

107. Ibid., I, 7.
108. Ibid., I, 8.

would not speak, yet people would receive something just by watching him and would say, "I feel contented and happy." This is the effect of a Siddha's company; this is why God can be attained through the grace of a saint or a Siddha. Such a being is the image of God.

However, it is difficult for you to understand this. Instead, you wander around without inhibition, under the control of your ego. As long as you continue to seek, you are far from your destination. By seeking, you lose. The more you desire to attain That, the farther you move away from it. All your efforts are in vain; rather than victory, you gain only defeat. But when there is total defeat, the ego melts and then the true hour of victory in the conquest of God begins. You see the effulgence of the natural state; your victory is the attainment of God. Otherwise, what is the meaning of victory? Ordinary victory is the victory of the ego, the victory of ignorance, in which the more you gain, the more difficulties you have to face.

Your problem is that you continue to exist. When will that fortunate day arrive when you become no one, when no one belongs to you, when you cease to exist? When will that hour come? At that time, there will be utter stillness and no image in the temple within. No form or sound will arise. There will be absolute silence, for there will be no one to speak and no one to hear. If that day comes, your fortune will blossom. At that very moment, you will be ready, and the grace of the Guru and the blessings of God will be showered upon you. Truly, at the moment when you and the world no longer exist, you will become worthy of receiving God's *prasad*.

Kabir wrote, "As long as I was looking for You, I did not see You. I went from door to door knocking, yet none of the doors was Yours. I looked for You on so many paths, yet none of them led to Your court. But when I received Ramananda's grace, when Guru Ramananda erased me and I became completely pure, I saw that You were behind me like my shadow. Wherever I went, You were there before me."

The Awareness of So'ham

The ego is a wall between oneself and God. A mind that is filled with ego wants to win God. Actually, almost everyone is looking not for God, but for religion. A person who seeks religion is in reality very egotistical; a religious person has religious pride, and for that reason it is very difficult to find humility, simplicity, or candor in him. But he is egotistical only because he has not completely attained the goal of religion. There is a saying: "A full pot makes no sound." When a pot is completely full, the liquid inside it remains noiseless. In the same way, when a person becomes perfect, ego is no more.

Any imperfection in a *sannyasi*, a *sadhu*, or a yogi is a sign of ego. If one has ego it dominates one's work in every field, whether one is a writer, a lecturer, or a spiritual guide. In their teachings, such beings always counsel humility, but they themselves never learn it. Their own egos are boundless. When four *sadhus* live together, their constant inner *japa* is, "Who is going to be the boss? How can I make myself more respected than anyone else?" In this way, their egos are fed instead of weakened.

A scripture says:

eka eva mahānātmā so'hankāro'bhidhīyate,
sa jīvaha so'ntarātmeti gīyate tattva chintakaihi.

Only the Lord of the Self is great. He is called *ahamkara*, the pure ego. Knowers of the Truth call Him *jivatma*, the individual soul, and *antaratma*, the inner Self. When one fully understands that *aham*, or "I," and merges it into *so'ham*, one recognizes the Truth instantly.

vibheda-janake ajnāne nāshamātyantikam gate,
ātmāno brahmano bhedām asantam kaha karishyati.

In this verse of the *Vishnu Purana*, it is said that when the ignorance of one who sees duality is completely destroyed, the difference between that individual soul and the Supreme

Self becomes unreal forever. The root cause of this duality is our ego, our ignorance.

People of different religions never cease to fight. But think—is religion just another branch of the military? Why was religion created—to increase love among people or to make the fires of hatred blaze? The purpose of religion is to bring about social unity, to help us achieve universal brotherhood, to inspire us to work together with mutual love, and to enable us to reach God. But how do we practice it? We hate other religions as well as our fellow beings. In the *Vishnu Sahasranam*, which is contained in the *Mahabharata*, Bhishmacharya speaks about true religion:

esha me sarvadharmānām dharmō'dhikatamo mataha,
yadbhaktyā pundarīkāksham satvairarchennaraha sadā. [109]

He says that of all religions in which there is formal worship, he considers to be the greatest that religion in which God is worshipped through the singing of hymns, chanting, and absorption in devotion and faith. Any religion which teaches that God dwells in the heart lotus and in which He is reverently worshipped through *so'ham* and *hamsa* is great.

Truly, the entire world is God's. People have created distinctions among religions, but God has never done that. Members of different religious sects may say, "You do not belong to my religion, so I do not accept you." But God cannot do that. God cannot banish anyone from His kingdom, because He exists everywhere; there is no place in this universe that does not belong to Him. Therefore, if a religion does not include everyone, it cannot be God's religion.

The true religion is that in which one becomes aware of one's own Self. That Self is Consciousness, which nothing can surpass. Because it pervades everywhere, Consciousness must accept all; it cannot reject anyone. The religion of Con-

---

109. *Vishnu Sahasranam,* 10.

sciousness is God's true religion. It is the awareness of *ham-sa*, of "I am That," which is alive within everyone. For this reason, one should pursue the *hamsa* awareness with the understanding that all people are equal. To perform this worship of the Self is to revere the Lord of the heart. This is the natural state, which can also be called natural *samadhi*. Natural *samadhi* is God-realization. The truth is that God can be attained without any special *sadhana*. You want to attain Him, but you have already attained Him. You are trying to find Him, but you have already found Him. You are unaware of this. A person searching for his own Self is like a fish in the ocean searching for the ocean or a bird flying in the sky searching for the sky. After you attain God, you will realize that your search for God was a delusion.

First give up the delusion of seeking and then rid yourself of your ego. Root out anger and approach the Guru. God is in front of you and behind you, so you do not have to attain Him; you merely have to remember Him. Kabir, Nanak, Dadu, Jnaneshwar, Ekanath, and Tukaram all used a priceless word: Remember. You must remember your own Self. All these great beings said that it would be possible to find God only if you had lost Him. How can you lose God? God is your own Self, which exists naturally and spontaneously within you. He is the life of your life. He is always with you. Kabir wrote:

Mōkō kahān dhūndhe bande?
Mai tō tere pās me, mai tō tere pās me.
Na devāl me na masjid me,
Na kāshi kailāsa me.
Mōkō kahān dhūndhe bande?
Mai tō tere pās me.

Where are you looking for Me, My servant?
I am with you, I am with you.
Not in the temple, not in the mosque,
Not in Kashi or Kailas.

Where are you looking for Me, My servant?
I am with you.

This is the truth. This is why to attain the Self you need nothing but the grace of a holy being, a saint, or a Guru. Be careful—in natural yoga and natural *samadhi*, even trying to think of God is a hindrance. You may repeat, "Ram, Ram," and your effort will not go to waste. But when Ram is everywhere, who will repeat His name? When only Ram exists everywhere, what will be repeated? The yoga of Guru's grace is natural yoga, in which there is nothing to do. Simply attain Him and become serene. What does the God within you say? He says, "I am, I am." Listen to that for a while. The sound "I am that I am" always emanates from inside you. This is the sound that you should remember: *so'ham-hamsa.*

I once read a story by Tolstoy. A man had contracted a disease, and because people feared that it was contagious he was banished to a broken-down shack outside the village. There he lived for twenty-five years, supporting himself on the coins and scraps of food thrown his way by passersby. When at last he died, the villagers cremated his body and burned his belongings and clothing. Fearing that the germs of the disease had penetrated the earth, the doctors ordered the area under his hut to be dug up and burned as well. While the villagers were digging, they were amazed to discover a large treasure chest of pearls, diamonds, rubies, and other gems. The beggar had been sitting on top of millions of dollars, yet had been begging for pennies. He had not realized what was beneath him.

We are all like that beggar. The light of the universe is within us, but are we aware of it? Yoga exists naturally in our lives because the world is the embodiment of yoga. There is nothing to be done; all that is necessary is understanding. You have already found Him. You yourself are that which you are seeking; you seek only because you do not know your Self. If your destination were far away, there would be

some need to search for it, but you are standing right on top
of it. Remember this — the treasure lies beneath your very
seat. Kabir wrote:

ānkh na mūndau kān na rūndhau tanik kashta nahi dharanu,
khule naina pahichanaun hansi hansi sundar rūpa nihāranu.

"I see Him without closing my eyes, without plugging my
ears, without troubling my body. With great joy, I see His
beautiful form." Why should Kabir have closed his eyes? He
saw only Ram. Whatever he heard was the mantra, the
matruka shakti. His was the perfect understanding of one who
possesses the revolutionary eye of knowledge. The Truth is
always the Truth. There is beauty in every man and woman
in the world. Therefore, with your eyes open, lovingly and
joyfully perceive the Supreme Truth. The world is the play of
bliss.

The *Shiva Sutras* say, *lokānanda samādhi sukham*[110]—"The
bliss of the world is the ecstasy of *samadhi*." When you see
God's face pervading everyone, the bliss of *samadhi* arises.
The awareness of equality is the nectar of love. Drink that.
What ambrosia!

Kabir wrote, "I live in *unmani*, the state beyond the mind."
The word *unmani* is very significant. It describes the mind
which has turned within and in which all mental activity has
ceased. However, even in that state, Kabir used to weave
cloth and blankets and carry out all his other work. You need
not worry—if you transcend the mind, you will not become
mentally ill. The mind of a mentally diseased person has not
turned within, but has broken down because it has been
thinking so fast. It is exactly the opposite of a great being's
mind. *Unmani*, the indrawn mental state, is directed toward
the Self. Kabir wrote, "When my mind departed, I became
established in my own center." This is how holy men,
enlightened beings, and Gurus live.

---

110. *Shiva Sutras*, I, 18.

The Therapy Course

Like Kabir, one should find one's Self without giving up one's home. Nowadays it has become the custom for everyone to do *sadhana*. People follow so many practices and *sadhanas* and observe so many disciplines, yet never think with subtle understanding about what they are doing. Most of the time, they are in the same situation as Nasrudin.

Once Nasrudin left home for four days. When he returned people asked him, "Where have you been?"

"I was taking a therapy course," replied Nasrudin.

A friend asked, "How many of these courses are you going to take?"

"As many as possible," Nasrudin answered. "What can I do? I'm trying to find out which course will help me."

Use your eyes and ears to look and listen properly. Use your mind to think and contemplate correctly. With God's help, make decisions with your intellect. Do this so that in a single course you can rid yourself of the exhaustion created by all your other courses. Then, even if you do not attain the Truth, at least you will know what it is. The Truth dwells in everyone at all times; if it did not, it would not be the Truth. The course in meditation and right understanding is all you need in order to know that the Truth is always with you.

You continually watch what others are doing. "That person does it," you say to yourself, "so I want to do it, too." But you should first try to understand why someone else does what he does and whether it applies to you.

Once Mullah Nasrudin went to a mosque to do *namaj*. While everyone was bowing down, he suddenly tugged on the shirttail of the man in front of him. The man turned around and asked, "What are you doing?"

"Ask the person behind me," Nasrudin said. "He pulled on my shirt, so I thought that this must be customary in your mosque."

Actually, Nasrudin's shirttail had been caught up in the back, and the man behind him had pulled it down simply to make it look correct. Nasrudin had in turn tugged on the shirt of the man in front of him and, when asked why he did it, could only say, "Ask the person behind me." We all have the same habit. We never think independently about what we are doing.

The Process of Awakening

You must wake up from your dream. The state you call your waking state is not the true waking state. Ponder this a bit: When you are happy in your life, you think that it is real. Then you behave as you might if you were sleeping and someone were trying to awaken you. You say, "Wait a minute! I am having a beautiful dream, and I don't want to wake up until it is over."

Mullah Nasrudin was sound asleep, having a wonderful dream. His wife was trying to awaken him. "Wait!" the *mullah* said. "Not right now—there's still time." Again his wife tried to awaken him. "Wait!" he told her. "Not now!"

A moment later she tried again. This time the *mullah* was furious. "You have ruined everything!" he cried. "In my dream, a man was giving me a lot of money. I was filling a bag with coins and insisting on getting the full amount owed to me. But you were so stupid, woman, that without thinking you woke me up just at that moment. When I closed my eyes again, the *rupees* were gone and I couldn't find the man no matter where I looked. I was waiting for him to return, but you didn't give me enough time. Again you forced me to wake up. If you had only waited, I would have been incredibly fortunate!"

This is your way: When you are having a pleasant dream, you have no desire to wake up, and thus you get into the habit of dreaming more and more dreams. But remember this—whether they are joyful or painful, all dreams are the same, because once you wake up they no longer exist. It is

futile to hope for the attainment of joy through your dreams.
Unreality has no value; it is only a means of devaluing life.
   The great being Brahmananda said:

jāg re nara jāg pyāre ab to gāfil jāg re,
svapna jaise jāl rachnā kilā duniyā bhāg re,
dekh lo nija rūp tero guru charan anurāg re.

"O man, wake up! O dear one, wake up! O servant, wake up!
Run away from the world, which is like the net of a dream.
See your own Self. Love the Guru's feet." You must awaken
from the darkness of mundane life, which is like a profound
slumber. There is only one way to rouse yourself from this
interminable sleep, and that is to see your own Self. Kabir
wrote, *sadguru alakh jagāyā*—"The Sadguru has revealed the
invisible to me." Through the Guru's grace, awake to the
remembrance of your own Self. Life is composed of the petty
desires of worldliness and nothing more; do not become
involved in them.
   Whatever you do, do it consciously. Do not lose your
awareness. The day will certainly come when you will awake
to the Self, and then the entire world will be illumined.
Actually, it is already illumined, but when you attain that
light you will experience it as your own.
   If you truly perceive and experience pain, if you befriend it
and examine it closely, you will thank God as much for pain
as for joy. But if you do not have the right view of pain, you
will complain not only about pain, but about happiness as
well. A great Sufi saint said, "Unless you pass through pain,
you will not achieve happiness." A person who has not seen
the blackness of night can never see the light of day. That
light is concealed behind night's darkness; therefore, be
thankful for night. A perfect life is one in which there is no
complaining. When all complaining ceases, the mind becomes utterly pure and surrenders completely to the Self.
   If you do not observe self-control in *sadhana*, you might as
well give up the desire to attain the goal. Knowledge alone

can do nothing for you. And, although meditation is necessary, by itself it cannot help you achieve anything. In order to make the mind mindless, you must give up your chronic habits, which are the cause of your troubles and therefore of your complaints.

In yoga, meditation, worship, prayer, and all other spiritual techniques, you must begin by looking within. This is the significance of these practices. Make your Self manifest, talk to your Self, and remember not to let your mind wander here and there, even momentarily. Do not make it easy for your mind to harbor strange fantasies. Do not be its accomplice; do not listen to its instructions. If the flow of thoughts ceases even briefly, if the waves of the mind stop for just a moment, God will instantly manifest within. Now you keep wandering, but when you become free of thoughts you will find Him without searching. You will become one with Him.

You will have to work hard to free yourself from thinking, because the mind is ancient and is trapped in the meshes of habit. The mind has become one with its habits, and it must be set free.

Mullah Nasrudin had the habit of drinking, and his wife was always finding reasons for him to give it up. Once she brought him a newspaper article citing evidence of the harmful effects of drinking. "Look at this," she said. "An internationally renowned doctor reported in a recent lecture that many diseases are caused by drinking. Drinking creates so much trouble!"

"Bah! This is just rumor, just propaganda," Nasrudin assured her. "I've been drinking for so long, and all that ever happens when I'm drunk is that I fall into the gutter or go to sleep on the sidewalk. Drinking itself is my only disease. I'm telling you this from my own experience."

"But the doctors say that people who drink lose ten years of their life," she insisted.

"My death is far away," replied Nasrudin. "When it comes, then I'll take care of my drinking problem. As long as

I'm alive, I'll keep on drinking every day. Don't mention such things to me again."

"How can you be sure that you will stop drinking after you die?" his wife asked. "Your drinking habit is so deeply ingrained that I think you will keep drinking even after death!"

Like Nasrudin, you are always pursued by your habits. The strength of your mind ties you to old habits and makes you merge with them, so that it becomes impossible to tell the difference between you and your habits. Because you have become one with your habits, they follow you lifetime after lifetime. However, if you make the right kind of effort, you can certainly become free of them.

For example, suppose you have the habit of believing that you are old and now want to rid yourself of it. The only way to do this is to become completely absorbed in every task you perform. You must stop your mind from wandering here and there. If it begins to wander to a place ten miles away and you try hard to stop it, it may at first go only nine miles. The next time you try, it may go only eight miles. Eventually it will go only one mile, and finally the day will come when it will remain completely still.

The State of Absorption

You should keep up your efforts at *sadhana*. Let an intoxication arise so that the mind can become absorbed in the inner sound. At such times of absorption, even if some mishap occurs directly in front of you, you will not be affected. No calamity can touch you when the mind is absorbed. At that time, when you are face to face with the Self, when there is no place for the mind to run and no way for it to think, the death of the mind becomes certain. O friend, surrender the sword of the mind to the Self. The moment you give in, everything you have been longing for will take place. Wherever you go, you will find celestial gardens and you will be in bliss. Wherever you look, you will see the face of the Self. Whatever you drink will be the nectar of joy. Whatever sound you hear will be the music of the divine Self. Like a fish swimming in water, you will swim in the pervasion of divine Consciousness. The entire cosmos will be seen as the Self; wherever you go, you will find your own Self.

The river worries, "What will happen to me if I lose myself in the ocean?" But the river is deluded; its fears of being obliterated are groundless. If it gives itself up to the ocean, it will live forever. The river is afraid that it will lose everything, but in fact when it merges into the ocean it will become the ocean. When its limited individuality is erased, how joyful it will become! When the banks that bind it and make it small are destroyed, how great it will be! Once its existence as a river has been erased, it will never again know birth or death. But before that happens, it is afraid to give up the banks that hem it in, fearing that it will lose its form, its name, its individual existence, and its identity.

The mind is like this fearful river, and the Self, Consciousness, is the ocean. If you glimpse the Self even briefly and try to lose yourself in it, you will become fearless and able to stand firmly on your own feet.

In all situations, let *so'ham* arise within. That sound is the self-existent inner speech of the Self, and it is completely true and natural. Penetrate deeply into that sound. It is pointless to remain on the surface, to repeat God's name superficially while clouds continue to form within. You should become so absorbed in repeating the mantra that even if you are in a situation that would normally cause great pain, like having an operation, you will not be aware of any suffering.

Once the king of Kashi was to undergo a lengthy and dangerous appendectomy, which would naturally be very painful. Since the king had sworn never to take any kind of drug, his doctor was in a dilemma: Unless he made the king unconscious by giving him an anesthetic, how could he perform the operation? The king told the doctor, "Don't worry. Give me Lord Krishna's *Shri Bhagavad Gita*, which I recite every day, and I will chant it while you perform the operation." The doctor did not trust the king, for no operation had ever before been performed under such conditions. The king's abdomen would have to remain open for a long time; suppose his absorption in the chant were broken? The doctor decided to test the king first. "Alright," he told him, "chant the *Gita*." Then he began to prick the king's hands and legs with needles and knives. Not for a moment was the king's absorption disturbed by any trace of pain; he went on lovingly chanting the *Gita*. The doctor performed the appendectomy, and the king was not even aware that he was having an operation.

Such events can occur in an ordinary person's life as well. If a child is playing hockey and injures his foot, he can be so absorbed in the game that even though the foot is bleeding, he keeps running without realizing that he is hurt. This is the miracle of a one-pointed mind. When one becomes absorbed in *so'ham*, one is aware of neither the body nor the world. To become absorbed means to forget everything else, to become so immersed that nothing else remains. This is the state of true understanding. When one is absorbed in the mantra, the mind itself becomes mantra. There is an aphorism in the *Shiva Sutras* that describes this state: *chittam mantraha*[111]— "The mind is mantra."

During his operation, the king of Kashi, intoxicated from chanting the *Bhagavad Gita*, had risen above body-consciousness. Although he was in the body, he was separate from it. This is the state in which the Truth dwells; the scriptures say that pain cannot reach the Supreme Truth.

In the *Bhagavad Gita* the Lord tells Arjuna:

mantrā-sparshāstu kaunteya shītoshna-sukha-duhkhadāhā,
āgamāpāyino 'nityās tans titīkshasva bhārata.[112]

---

111. Ibid., II, 1.
112. *Bhagavad Gita*, II, 14.

"The contacts of the senses with their objects, O son of Kunti, which cause heat and cold, pleasure and pain, have a beginning and an end. They are impermanent. Endure them bravely, O Arjuna." The Lord explains that pain and pleasure are the inherent nature of the four psychic instruments.[113] They come and go; pleasure can become pain, and pain pleasure. If one is patient and rises above them, one will reach a state in which one experiences neither pleasure nor pain. The toil of reading the scriptures reaches only the physical and subtle bodies. Beyond these is the *turiya* state, the supracausal body. This is one's true nature, one's own ocean.

One's meditation should merge in the space between *so* and *ham*; no fraction of the mind should remain. Only when the mind stops wandering can one be certain that one has become absorbed in God. When one achieves this absorption, one feels that one has suddenly fallen into the ocean of God. There is nowhere to go and no *sadhana* left to follow. One's Siddhahood becomes perfect. This is true surrender; it is the gateway to the Truth.

The Secret Ray of Love

When two people are genuinely in love, they sit very still. Because their love is true, it is free of desire and beyond the senses. True lovers want nothing but to be close to each other; their highest joy is to sit in inner absorption. They do not want to ruin that joy by talking, for they know that if they move or speak, their priceless moments of closeness will slip through their fingers. A feeling such as this is like mercury— if it slips and falls, it disperses. Therefore, true lovers sit together quietly. They do not even say, "I love you," because that is useless chatter. When there is genuine love, there is

---

113. The mind, subconscious mind, intellect, and ego.

no idle talk. Talking begins only when love is lost; then one has to keep saying, "I love you," merely to inspire trust.

Many people become angry with me out of love. They say, "Baba didn't look at me," or "Baba hasn't spoken to me for a month," or "When Baba looked at me, he didn't smile." People who say these things do not understand that when I sit on my chair I look at everyone once, silently and with great joy. That is truly welcoming people; that is loving them. To say, "I love you," is not love, but merely an imitation of love. True love has no language. If I look at someone once, silently emitting a ray of love, that is sublime. This is true and should be understood: Love is a secret ray of the eyes.

There are people to whom I do not speak year after year; others point this out to them. But those who do this are foolish and fail to understand the nature of our relationship. The relationship of love is a silent one. An egotistical person is hurt if Baba does not speak to him, but there is no need to speak. To see everyone once is sufficient.

Once a Moslem priest asked Rabi'a Basri, "Does God speak to you?"

Rabi'a answered, "Does one have to talk to God? I keep looking at Him, and He keeps looking at me. What could be more sublime? Seeing Him, I become utterly content, and then He is happy with me. What could be more wonderful than perfect contentment?"

What can one achieve through conversation? Love for God arises spontaneously. It does not come through fear, greed, the desire for praise, or any kind of activity. It cannot be had for the asking. When a person keeps watching God, he obtains the right outlook in his life. Then his own vision becomes *darshan*, and wherever he looks he sees God. Therefore, Kabir wrote, "Anything is good when it is true, but even love is unacceptable when it is false." Truth never takes a person on a false path; only falsehood makes one go astray. One should love God for the sake of love.

You have never experienced the true prayer, which culminates in the stirring of love. Most people find prayer bitter because they pray out of fear, to escape hell, or to obtain fame and honor. That is not real prayer. Real prayer is directed toward the Self.

Mullah Nasrudin's friend was dying. He was a priest who, throughout his life, had been very religious and had spent a great deal of time in prayer. Because the head priest of the village was out of town, only Nasrudin was there to perform the last rites. Nasrudin stared at his friend and said, "Since your last hour has come, I will start praying at once, without wasting any time." He began to shout, "O Allah! O Satan!"

An onlooker asked, "What are you doing?"

The *mullah* replied, "Who knows whether this man is going to Allah or to the Devil? Because it is the final hour, there isn't time to decide which one to address. I thought I had better pray to both of them, so that everything will be taken care of no matter where he goes."

Most of the time, your prayers are like those of the *mullah*. Since love for God has not arisen in you, your praying is calculated. However, the correct way to pray is to surrender yourself.

The Six Vices

A person should always cultivate pure qualities. He should develop virtues not only to attain the Self but to experience joy in his worldly life as well. In the *Bhagavad Gita* Lord Krishna says:

dambho darpo'bhimānashcha krodhaha pārushyameva cha,
ajñānam chābhijātasya pārtha sampadamāsurīm. [114]

"Ostentation, arrogance, conceit, anger, harshness, and ignorance belong to one who is born with a demoniacal

---

114. *Bhagavad Gita*, XVI, 4.

nature, O Arjuna." In *Jnaneshwari*, Jnaneshwar Maharaj elaborates the verse above as follows:

Krishna said, "O Arjuna, ego is the root of all defects. One of the demoniacal qualities is ostentation. O Arjuna, even if a man's mother is as pure and worthy of worship as a holy place, if he brings her naked into the public eye it will bring about his degradation. Although the Guru's teachings grant the desired fruit, to shout them at the crossroads brings harm. Although a boat is the means by which we cross a river, if we tie that boat on top of our heads when we are drowning, it will bring about our death. It is well known that food sustains life, but if we eat too much of it for the sake of its delicious taste, it will become poison for us and create disease. Similarly, even though religion is our support in this world as well as in the next, if we proudly proclaim our observance of it, the same religion that brings salvation will become a source of evil. Therefore, O Arjuna, religion becomes irreligion when we openly discuss our religiosity in public, making a display of our pious actions. This kind of action is ostentation.

"Now hear the characteristics of arrogance. When a fool acquires a smattering of knowledge or reads a few scriptures, he begins to criticize the scholars. When a horse is whipped up by its rider and begins to gallop, it regards even Airavata, the elephant of heaven, as insignificant. A chameleon that climbs to the top of a thorny bush considers heaven to be low. The flames of a grass-fed fire rise to the sky, and a fish swimming in a pond or a lake scorns the ocean. In the same way, a man becomes arrogant about his wife, his wealth, his learning, his reputation, and his standing among others. A beggar feels proud of the day's meal that he gets from the house of another. An unfortunate man tears down his hut when he is protected by the shadow of the clouds and breaks his water pot when he sees a mirage. Similarly, when a man is full of conceit because of his worldly possessions, he is entrapped by arrogance.

"Now hear the characteristics of pride. Everyone believes in the Vedas. The Supreme Being should be worshipped with faith. As the sun, He is the only giver of light to the world. Everyone desires to rise to the throne of an emperor, and all people wish for freedom from death. So it should not be suprising if everyone praises God and feels devotion to Him because of these gifts. But envy arises in the mind of a wicked person when he hears God praised. As the creeper of his envy flourishes he says, 'I will swallow up your God. I will poison your Vedas; I will destroy them with my power.' When a moth sees a flame, it becomes agitated. A firefly dislikes the sun, and to the *titavi* bird the ocean is an enemy. In the same way, a man who is trapped in his own pride cannot bear the name of God. He behaves like a stepson with his own father, afraid that his father will get a share of his wealth. A person who is inflated with ego and filled with pride should be considered to be on the road to hell.

"O Arjuna, now I will explain the characteristics of anger. Other people's joy tastes as bitter as poison to a wicked person, and he becomes angry when he sees another's pleasure. When water is sprinkled into hot oil, the oil crackles furiously. When a jackal sees the moon, it burns in agitation. The sinful owl loses its eyesight when the bright sun, which lights the entire world, rises in the morning. Daybreak, the joy of humankind, is more painful than death for thieves. Milk becomes poison when it enters the stomach of a snake. Instead of cooling down, the great fire beneath the sea burns more fiercely because of the limitless water of the ocean. To become increasingly enraged at the sight of others' learning, happiness, and good fortune is called anger.

"Now I will explain to you the characteristics of harshness. The mind of a harsh person is a viper's nest. His look is as scathing as the shot of an arrow. His speech is like a shower of scorpions. All his actions are as jagged as the blade of a saw. He is so caustic within and without that he is the lowest of all men. This is a description of harshness.

"Now hear the characteristics of ignorance. A stone is unable to distinguish between the sensations of heat and cold. A person born blind cannot tell the difference between day and night. A blazing fire consumes everything without distinction. The philosophers' stone cannot differentiate between iron and gold. Although a ladle is dipped into various kinds of food, it does not taste any of them. The wind does not know the difference between straight and crooked. In the same way, an ignorant person cannot determine which actions are right and which are wrong, or what is pure and what is impure. He combines both sin and virtue and eats them, just as a child puts whatever he finds into his mouth without knowing whether it is good or bad for him. His state is so deplorable that his intellect cannot even distinguish the sweet from the bitter. This state is called ignorance. There is no doubt about this.

"I have explained to you the characteristics of the six vices. No matter how small the body of a serpent is, it contains venom. The three fires of the day of doom seem to be insignificant in number, but if these fires were to burst into flame, the whole world would not suffice as an oblation. In the same way, there are only six of these vices, but when they come together the force of evil acquires great strength. If the three bodily humors unite in the body, one cannot find refuge from death even if one clings to the feet of Brahman. But these six vices are twice as evil as the humors. The structure of evil stands on the foundation of the six vices. They are never weak. If all the harmful planets were to come into conjunction in the same sign of the zodiac, if all the sins were to assail a slanderer, if many diseases were to attack a man doomed to die, if all bad omens were to meet at an inauspicious moment, if a man whom one trusted without reservation turned out to be a thief, or if an exhausted man were thrown into a flood, that would be the effect of the six vices. A person under their influence commits atrocities. When the life of a goat is about to end, a scorpion with seven stingers attacks it. In the same way, the six vices sting a man. When he approaches the path of liberation, he cries out, "I will not walk on this path!" and plunges into worldly affairs. He descends into lower and lower births and eventually reaches the lowest order of inanimate objects. In him all six vices unite and strengthen the force of evil. Thus, I have described the characteristics of the six vices."[115]

The next verse of the *Bhagavad Gita* is:

daivī sampadvimokshāya nibandhāyāsurī matā,
mā shuchaha sampadam daivīmabhijāto'si pāndava.[116]

"The divine nature leads to liberation, and the demoniacal to bondage. Grieve not, O Arjuna; you were born with divine qualities." Jnaneshwar's commentary continues:

"The first of these two, the divine nature, should be considered the dawn of the sun of liberation. But the demoniacal qualities form the iron chain of infatuation which binds. Do not be frightened as you listen to these words. O Arjuna, why should day be frightened of night? Only those who allow the six vices to dwell in them are bound by evil. But, O Arjuna, you are virtue incarnate. Therefore, O Partha, become the master of divine qualities and attain the joy of ultimate liberation.

"Ornaments are made in different shapes, yet the gold in them always remains unchanging. In the same way,

---

115. *Jnaneshwari*, XVI, 215-262.
116. *Bhagavad Gita*, XVI, 5.

this play of various beings is created, undergoes many changes, assumes many forms, and is finally destroyed, yet the Self that exists in all of them is imperishable. He who sees that the principle of the Self is apart from the individual soul and yet no different from it is the most perceptive among seers. Such a one is very fortunate."[117]

The Self and the Body

samam pashyan hi sarvatra samavasthitamīshvaram,
na hinastyātmanātmanam tato yāti parām gatim.[118]

"Because he who sees the same Lord dwelling equally everywhere does not destroy the Self by his individuality, he goes to the highest goal."

"This body is a vessel containing the *gunas* and the senses, the threefold mixture of the bodily humors, and the collection of the five elements. It is hideous. It is like a scorpion with five stingers, or a fierce fire blazing in five different directions, or a ferocious lion in the form of the soul who has come upon the lair of a deer. Living in such a body, who will stab the belly of the transitory with the knife of knowledge of the eternal and thus become free of cares?

"O Arjuna, a man of knowledge dwells in this body without harming the Self. Then, when the body falls away, he merges into the principle of the Self. Having passed through thousands of lives, yogis plunge into this union through the power of their knowledge and yogic practice, knowing that they will never return. That state lies on the farther shore of the river of this created universe of beings, names, and forms. It is the birthplace of the transcendental state, even beyond the boundary of the

---

117. *Jnaneshwari*, XVI, 263-268.
118. *Bhagavad Gita*, XIII, 28.

divine sound; it is the Supreme Brahman. Liberation and
the supreme state come to rest there, just as all rivers
merge into the ocean. The joy and bliss of that attainment
come of their own accord to wash the feet of those beings
who banish duality from their minds and behave equally
with everyone, seeing the Self in all. Just as there is only
one light in all lamps, so God, who is without beginning,
is equally present in all. O Arjuna, one who lives with the
perception of unity is never bound by birth and death.
Therefore, I praise again and again the fortunate being
whose vision is always firm in equality-awareness."[119]

prakrutyaiva cha karmāni kriyamānāni sarvashaha,
yah pashyati tathā'tmānamakartāram sa pashyati. [120]

"One who sees that all actions are performed by the natural
forces alone, and that the Self is actionless, truly sees."

"An enlightened being knows that all the actions that
proceed from the powers of action, the senses of perception, the mind, and the intellect are performed by the
natural force [*prakruti*]. Such a being knows that it is the
people who live in a house who perform actions; the
house itself does nothing. Clouds pass through the sky as
they please, but the sky itself neither moves nor sways. In
the same way, *prakruti*, animated by the light of the Self,
sports in various ways according to the three *gunas*, while
the Self remains uninvolved in the sport, indifferent as a
pillar. A being who has seen the light of knowledge
through his firm understanding of this truth has truly
realized the Self, which is free from doership."[121]

yadā bhūtaprithagbhāvamekasthamanupashyati,
tata eva cha vistāram brahma sampadyate tadā. [122]

---

119. *Jnaneshwari,* XIII, 1063-1073.
120. *Bhagavad Gita,* XIII, 29.
121. *Jnaneshwari,* XIII, 1074-1077.
122. *Bhagavad Gita,* XIII, 30.

"When a man sees all varieties of beings as resting in the One and spreading forth from That alone, he then becomes Brahman."

"O Arjuna, when a person no longer sees the diversity in all these forms, all forms are seen as one and he understands them all to be the Absolute. Just as there are waves in water, atoms and grains in the earth, rays in the sun, limbs in the body, various feelings in the mind, and different sparks in fire, all these beings and forms belong to the same Self. When one perceives this with the vision of knowledge, one acquires the ship of the wealth of the Absolute. Then, wherever one looks, one sees Brahman and attains limitless love.

"O Arjuna, I have explained to you the nature of matter [prakruti] and spirit [purusha] and have shown them to you step by step. You should value this knowledge as though you had obtained a handful of nectar or come upon a hidden treasure. You have attained supreme worthiness. But, O Arjuna, as long as you do not experience this completely, you will not have firm conviction in your mind. I will tell you one or two important things, but first pay attention and listen to me."

After saying this, Shri Krishna began to speak further. Arjuna made his mind very attentive and began to listen to Him. [123]

anāditvān nirgunatvāt paramātmāyamavyayah,
sharīrastho'pi kaunteya na karoti na lipyate. [124]

"Without beginning and without *gunas*, the imperishable Supreme Self, though dwelling in the body, O son of Kunti, neither acts nor becomes tainted."

Shri Krishna said, "O Arjuna, the nature of the Supreme Being is like the sun, which is reflected in water

---

123. *Jnaneshwari*, XIII, 1078-1082.
124. *Bhagavad Gita*, XIII, 31.

but does not get wet by contact with the water. The sun existed even before the water and will continue to exist after it. O Arjuna, only in the interim do others see it reflected in the water. It constantly remains as it is. In the same way, it is impossible to say that the Self exists in the body because it exists within itself everywhere. When a face is reflected in a mirror, people say that the face is in the mirror; similarly, it is said that the Self lives in the body. But it is entirely false to say that there is any contact between the body and the Self. How could one say that wind and sand can mix together? Could a rope tie fire to cotton? How could the sky be joined with a stone? The relationship between the body and the Self is like two travelers, one going east and another west, who meet somewhere along the path. The same relationship that exists between light and darkness, or between the living and the dead, exists between the body and the Self. The same difference exists between the body and the Self as exists between day and night, or gold and cotton. The body is a product of the five elements. Imprisoned in the bondage of actions, it spins around, tied to the wheel of birth and death. The body is like a lump of butter that is thrown into the fire of time and perishes in the split second it takes a fly to flap its wings. If it falls into the fire, it is reduced to ashes, if it falls into the hands of dogs and crows, it turns into excrement, and if neither of these things happens, it becomes a heap crawling with worms. O Arjuna, in whatever state the body may be, it is deplorable. This is the condition of the body.

"But the Self is beginningless, eternal, self-existent, and without attributes. It is neither whole nor divided, neither active nor inactive, neither subtle nor gross. Because it is formless, it cannot be said to be perceived or unperceived, shining or dark, small or large. It is the Void, yet it is neither empty nor full. It possesses nothing and lacks nothing. It neither has form nor is without form. It neither experiences bliss nor lacks it. It is neither one nor many, neither free nor bound, for it is the Self. Since it has no outer sign, it cannot be said to be this way or that. It is neither self-created nor made by another. It neither speaks nor is mute. It does not come into existence with the creation of the universe, nor is it destroyed with its dissolution, for it is the final resting place of both creation and destruction. It can be neither measured nor defined; it neither increases nor decreases; it is imperishable and inexhaustible, for it has no substance. When this is the nature of the Self, O friend Arjuna, to say that the Self lives in the body is like saying that space can be limited to the shape of a pot. The Self is all-pervasive; like the sky. Bodies form and dissolve, but the Self remains eternally the same. As day and night appear and disappear, so do bodies come and go through the power of the Self. Therefore, although the Self lives in the body, it neither acts nor causes action, nor has it anything to do with the actions that occur spontaneously. The nature of the Self is not subject to notions of greater or less. Although the Self is present in the body, it is untouched by the body's changes."[125]

yathā sarvagatam saukshmyādākāsham nopalipyate,
sarvatrāvasthito deha tathā'tmā nopalipyate.[126]

"Just as the all-pervasive ether [space] is not tainted because of its subtlety, so the Self that exists everywhere in the body suffers no stain."

"There is no place where space does not exist, yet the impurity of a place does not affect it. In the same way, the Self permeates all bodies and places, yet is never contaminated by their impurities. I am clarifying for you again and again the characteristics of the Self so that you will

---

125. *Jnaneshwari*, XIII, 1088-1113.
126. *Bhagavad Gita*, XIII, 32.

clearly understand that the knower of the field is different from the field.[127] When iron comes in contact with a magnet, it moves toward it but does not become the magnet. The same relationship exists between the field and the knower of the field. The light of a lamp makes it possible for activities to go on inside a house, but there is a great difference between the lamp and the house. O Arjuna, although fire is latent in wood, this does not mean that fire is wood. The knower of the field, the Self, should be regarded in the same way. A person who considers this matter very well comes to realize that the same difference exists between the knower of the field and the field as exists between the sky and its clouds or between the sun and a mirage."[128]

yathā prakāshayatyekah krutsnam lokamimam ravihi,
kshetram kshetrī tathā krutsnam prakāshayati bhārata. [129]

"Just as one sun illumines the entire world, so also the Lord of the field [the Supreme Self] illumines the entire field, O Bharata."

"Enough has been said about this. Just as the sun in the sky illumines the entire earth, so the knower of the field illumines the entire field. There is no longer any room for questions or doubts."[130]

The State of an Enlightened Being

It is important for us to understand how a being who is beyond the three *gunas* behaves with respect to them. How

---

127. In the thirteenth chapter of the *Bhagavad Gita,* Lord Krishna describes the relationship between the body and the Self by comparing them to a field and the knower of that field.
128. *Jnaneshwari,* XIII, 1114-1120.
129. *Bhagavad Gita,* XIII, 33.
130. *Jnaneshwari,* XIII, 1121-1122.

does he act in the world while maintaining the awareness of the Self? The teachings of the *Bhagavad Gita* are not intended to isolate people from the world. Seekers should know the way of life of a being who has transcended the three *gunas*. Now read the description of his characteristics.

nānyam gunebhyah kartāram yadā drashtānupashyati,
gunebhyashcha param vetti madbhāvam so'dhigacchati. [131]

"When the seer beholds no agent other than the *gunas* and knows that which is higher than them, he attains My being."

"Listen. Know that all three *gunas* reveal their own power, using the body as an instrument. Just as fire assumes the form of its fuel, the water of the earth appears in the form of a tree, milk is transformed into curds, and sweetness takes the form of sugarcane, similarly, the three *gunas*, along with the psychic instruments, take the form of the body and become the source of bondage. O Arjuna, it is remarkable that in spite of this close relationship between the three *gunas* and the body, still the individual soul does not lack even the slightest freedom. These three *gunas*, according to their inherent nature, have performed the accumulated past actions of the body as well as its current actions. Yet the Self, which is free of all attributes, is not diminished because of them.

"Now, because you are like a bee reveling in the lotus of knowledge, I will tell you how it is that an individual soul, although entangled in these three *gunas*, can easily attain liberation. This is the same principle I already explained to you; [132] the Self, although involved with the three *gunas*, is not of them. O Arjuna, when the individual soul realizes the Self, he understands this just as a person who awakens from sleep knows that a dream is an illusion.

"When one is sitting quietly on the bank of a river, one

---

131. *Bhagavad Gita*, XIV, 19.
132. In the beginning of the thirteenth chapter of the *Bhagavad Gita*.

understands that whatever is moving with the ripples is not one's body but a mere reflection. Just as an actor gives a skillful performance but does not become deceived by the role he is playing, an individual should know that he is different from the three *gunas*. The seasons are held by the sky, yet the sky does not allow itself to be affected by any illusion of difference in its own nature. In the same way, although the Self is amidst the three *gunas*, it remains separate and beyond them. That self-born Principle is always firm in the primordial seat of *aham brahmāsmi*—'I am Brahman.' Anchored in that seat, the Supreme Principle, the Self, says, 'I am the Witness; I am not the doer. It is the *gunas* that have created an army of actions.' Actions arise from the different characteristics of purity, activity, and inertia and are merely the modifications of these three *gunas*.

"How do I stand amidst the combination of these *gunas* and actions? Springtime in a forest is the source of all its beauty. When the sun rises, all the stars fade and vanish, the sun crystal gleams, the lotuses blossom, and the darkness is dispelled, but although these activities take place because of the sun's rising, the sun itself does not perform them. In the same way, although I am the cause of all actions, I am never their doer and actions do not affect Me. The *gunas* become manifest through Me. I give them power, and when they pass away, the attributeless, eternal Principle that remains is Myself. O Arjuna, one who is uplifted through his intellect and discrimination attains the supreme state and transcends the limitations of the *gunas*."[133]

gunānetānatītya trīn dehī deha samudbhavān,
janma-mrityu-jarāduhkhair vimukto'mritam-ashnute.[134]

---

133. *Jnaneshwari*, XIV, 278-297.
134. *Bhagavad Gita*, XIV, 20.

"The individual soul, having transcended the three *gunas* out of which the body is evolved, is freed from birth, death, decay, and pain and attains immortality."

"A being who has risen above all the *gunas* knows fully that independent Principle, for knowledge has been indelibly imprinted upon him. In short, O Arjuna, such an enlightened being becomes one with Me just as a river is absorbed into the ocean. Like a parrot that has escaped from its perch and sits freely on the branch of a tree, an enlightened being is freed from individuality and *maya* and becomes firm in the primordial 'I'-principle of *aham brahmāsmi*. O Arjuna, all this time he has been snoring in the deep sleep of ignorance, but now he awakens to the knowledge of his true nature. O Arjuna, bravest of the brave! When the mirror of delusion that creates duality falls from his hand, he can no longer see any reflection in it. When the wind of identification with the body ceases to blow, the individual soul and Shiva become one, just as waves merge into the ocean. As clouds dissolve into the sky at the end of the rainy season, so the individual soul merges into Brahman and becomes one with Me. After becoming identical with Brahman, he does not become involved with the *gunas*, which are born of the body, although he continues to live in the body until it perishes. As the light of a lamp does not diminish when it is covered with a glass shade, as the fire beneath the ocean cannot be extinguished by the ocean's waters, so his intelligence cannot be corrupted by the ebb and flow of the *gunas*. Although he appears to live in the body, he is unaffected by the nature of the body, just as the moon is reflected in water yet remains detached from it. All three *gunas*, through their own power, manifest the body as a disguise and make it dance. But an enlightened being does not allow himself to be aware of them even in a moment of forgetfulness. Not for an instant does he lose his consciousness of his identity with Brahman. The awareness of the Self becomes so firm in his heart that he is not conscious of performing actions in the body. When a serpent sheds its skin and enters its hole, it is no longer concerned with what will happen to the skin. When a lotus blossoms, its fragrance merges into the air and never returns to the lotus. In the same way, when such a being is united with Brahman, he is unaware of the nature of his body. Therefore, the six conditions, such as birth, old age, and death, affect only the body; they do not touch an enlightened being. When a clay pot is broken into fragments, it should be understood that the space inside the pot has merged with the vast space outside and has assumed its form. In the same way, when the identification with the body vanishes and the nature of the Self is remembered, what remains except the Self? Although he lives in the body, an enlightened being has the knowledge of the Self. That is why I say that he has transcended the three *gunas*."

Hearing these words of the Lord, Arjuna became as happy as a peacock when it hears a thunderclap. [135]

Lord Krishna continues to describe the state of an enlightened being:

". . . You must understand this mystery very clearly— the *gunas* operate through the power of the Self. The following analogies or examples can be given. The sun sets in motion all actions and activities, yet it quietly watches them all. When the moon rises, the ocean is at high tide, the moonstone exudes moisture, and the moon-lotus blossoms, yet the moon remains separate and detached from them all. Whether the wind blows forcefully or gently, the sky remains motionless and unchanging. Likewise, an enlightened being is not disturbed by contact with the *gunas*. O Arjuna, by the characteristics described above, recognize a being who has transcended the qualities. Now listen to the way he lives." [136]

---

135. *Jnaneshwari*, XIV, 298-317.
136. Ibid., XIV, 342-345.

samaduhkhasukhah svasthah samaloshtāshmakānchanaha,
tulyapriyāpriyo dhīrastulyanindātmasamstutihi. [137]

"He is the same in pleasure and pain. He dwells in the Self. To him a clod of earth, stone, and gold are alike; the dear and the unfriendly are the same. He is firm and remains the same in censure and praise."

"O Arjuna, in a garment there is nothing but thread inside and out. In the same way, an enlightened being perceives that the universe of the animate and inanimate is nothing but the Self. Just as God grants the same supreme state to His enemies as to His devotees, an enlightened being considers both pain and pleasure to be equal. In reality, as long as a person moves about like a fish in the water of worldly life, he dwells in the body and experiences pain and pleasure. But an enlightened being has completely renounced both pain and pleasure and is wholly absorbed in his true nature. When crops in the fields are harvested, the grain is separated from the husks. When a river relinquishes its current and merges into the ocean, its turbulence is left behind. Similarly, when a being delights in the Self, he is unaware of bodily pain or pleasure. Just as night and day are alike to a pillar, the pairs of opposites, such as gain and loss, pain and pleasure, are the same for a being who resides in the Self. It makes no difference to a sleeping man whether he is touched by the body of a celestial maiden or a serpent. Similarly, to a being who is absorbed in his own Self, the pairs of opposites that affect the body are equal. Therefore, from his point of view, there is no difference between gold and cow dung or a diamond and a rock. Whether the joy of heaven enters his house or a tiger attacks him, it does not affect his state of oneness with Brahman in the least. A dead man does not come back to life. A roasted

---

137. *Bhagavad Gita,* XIV, 24.

seed does not sprout. Similarly, the mental equilibrium of such a being is never disturbed. Whether someone showers him with praise by calling him Brahman or condemns him by calling him wretched, he is like ashes, which neither burn nor are extinguished. Just as in the abode of the sun there is neither darkness nor lamplight, so neither praise nor blame has any meaning for an enlightened being."[138]

mānāpamānayostulyas tulyo mitrāripakshayoho,
sarvārambhaparityāgī gunātītah sa uchyate.[139]

"He is the same in honor and dishonor and the same to friend and foe. He abandons all undertakings. He is said to have transcended the *gunas*."

"Whether he is worshipped as God or condemned as a thief, whether people surround him with bulls and elephants or make him a king, whether he is approached by friends or attacked by enemies, it is the same to him, just as for the light of the sun there is neither night nor day. The sky remains untouched by whichever of the six seasons approaches; in the same way, his mind is not troubled by disparity. There is one more characteristic of his behavior: He does not feel that he performs any action. He eliminates all actions, throws them aside, and destroys the root tendency that had driven him to act. Through the knowledge of his own Self, he himself becomes the fire in which all the fruits of his actions are burned to ashes. No desire for this world or the next arises in him. He accepts with indifference whatever comes to him easily and naturally. He is as unaffected by happiness or pain as if he were a stone, and his mind has abandoned thoughts and doubts. If you see this kind of behavior in a being, consider him one who has transcended the *gunas*."

---

138. *Jnaneshwari*, XIV, 346-358.
139. *Bhagavad Gita*, XIV, 25.

After this, Lord Shri Krishna said, "Now listen to the means through which an individual can transcend the *gunas*."[140]

True Devotion

mām cha yo'vyabhichārena bhaktiyōgena sevate,
sa gunān samatītyaitān brahmabhūyāya kalpate.[141]

"He who serves Me with unswerving devotion and crosses beyond the *gunas* is fit to become Brahman."

"O Arjuna, only he who serves Me with an unswerving mind through the path of devotion can burn up the *gunas*. I must explain all these things: who I am, the nature of devotion to Me, and the meaning of promiscuity. O Arjuna, I want to tell you that just as a jewel and its luster are one, in the same way I dwell in this universe. Just as water is in the netherworld, space in the sky, sweetness in sugar, flame in fire, a stalk in the lotus, branches and fruit on a tree, snow on the Himalayas, and curdled milk in yogurt, similarly, the universe is in Me. I am the universe. It is not necessary to strip the moon to know it. One can recognize *ghee* even if it is not heated and melted. Even if ornaments are not melted down, they are still gold. It is not necessary to unravel a piece of cloth to know that it is still thread, and one need not smash a pot to see that it is clay. In the same way, you do not have to destroy the sense of the universe before you can attain Me, for I am everything. To realize Me in this manner is to have single-hearted devotion. To have any sense of duality, any knowledge other than that of oneness, is promiscuity. Therefore, renounce the sense of difference, and with an

---

140. *Jnaneshwari*, XIV, 359-367.
141. *Bhagavad Gita*, XIV, 26.

undivided mind recognize Me as your own Self. Just as a gold ornament is not different from the gold in it, you should not regard the universe as different from your Self. A ray of light is one with that light, and all individuals are my rays. Just as there are atoms in the earth or snowflakes on mountain peaks, remember that your 'I' exists in Me. No matter how small a wave may be, it can never be different from the ocean. Similarly, there is no difference between Me and the Universal Self. The bliss that springs from the awareness and vision of oneness is that which I call devotion; it is the essence of all knowledge and yoga. That blissful vision of oneness is like the unbroken showers that make the rain clouds and the ocean appear as one.

"The sky and the air in the top of a well intermingle even though there is no apparent connection between them. In the same way, although there is no apparent connection between an enlightened being and the Absolute, they are one. Just as light streams uninterruptedly from the sun to its reflection, the awareness of *so'ham* extends from the individual to the Supreme Being. Once established in this awareness, a being spontaneously merges into God. When a grain of salt has melted in the ocean, the process of melting comes to an end. O Arjuna, after a fire has consumed grass, it burns out. Similarly, once the sense of duality is obliterated through knowledge, not even the memory of it remains. Any thought that God is on the farther shore and that the devotee is on this one is destroyed, and only their primordial and eternal unity remains. O Arjuna, once one savors union with Brahman, there is no longer any question of conquering the senses. O wise Arjuna, this state, which My devotees attain, is the nature of Brahman. Let Me tell you again: Whoever is devoted to Me while in this world will be served by the state of Brahman like a devoted wife. As the raging current of a river has no possible destination but the ocean, so one who serves Me with this enlightened vision adorns the state of Brahman. This state of total absorption in Brahman is called *sayujya* and is one of the four types of liberation. Service to Me is the *sadhana* for attaining the state of Brahman. But never think that I am just a means to that end. Because this thought may arise in your mind, I want you to know that Brahman is not different from Me."[142]

The Root of Wrong Action

Why does one follow the wrong path? What impels one to perform bad actions? Day after day people fall rather than improve, and this is a major problem. What does Jnaneshwar's commentary on the *Bhagavad Gita* say is the root of all sins? Arjuna asks a question about this:

atha kena prayukto'yam pāpam charati pūrushaha,
anicchannapi vārshneya balādiva niyojitaha.[143]

"But by what is a man impelled to commit sin, as if by force, even against his own will, O Krishna?"

"O Lord, how is it that even the wise fall from the state of the Self and, leaving the path, go astray? Why do even those who have become omniscient, who know what to accept and what to avoid, take on the duties of others and neglect their own? A blind man cannot discriminate between the grain and the husk, but why do even wise men sometimes become confused about what to accept and what to reject? Even those who are no longer confused about which actions to perform embrace the tumult of the world and remain unsatisfied, while those who go into seclusion return to live among people. If they were to remain hidden, they could escape evil, but they purposely perform sinful actions. A mind that dislikes an object

---

142. *Jnaneshwari*, III, 368-400.
143. *Bhagavad Gita*, III, 36.

thinks about it constantly, and if the mind is told not to do this, it is ready to fight. What is this tyrannical power which compels even the wise? O Krishna, please explain this to me."[144]

kāma esha krodha esha rajoguna-samudbhavaha,
mahāshano mahāpāpmā viddhyenam iha vairinam.[145]

"It is desire; it is anger born of the quality of passion, all-devouring, all-sinful. Know this to be the enemy here."

Then the highest of all beings, Shri Krishna, who dwells in the minds of desireless yogis, said, "Listen, O Arjuna, and I will tell you. O brother, desire and anger impel a person to act. They are without the slightest compassion. They are as cruel as death. They are serpents surrounding the wealth of knowledge, tigers in the ditch of sense objects, low killers on the path of devotion. They are rocks that endanger the fortress of the body; they are a wall encircling the village of the senses. Their power has spread throughout the entire world. They are the demons of the mantras of *rajoguna*, who live on the food of ignorance. In reality, they are born of *rajoguna*, but *tamoguna* is also fond of them and has invested them with its own negligence and infatuation. Because desire and anger suck one's life, they are highly regarded in the kingdom of death. When they are hungry, the entire universe is not a morsel large enough to satisfy them. They stretch out their hands farther as their expectations increase. Delusion, of whom they are very fond, is the younger sister of hope, and when she opens her palm and asks that something be put in it, the fourteen worlds are a mere trifle for her to grasp. Delusion is so extraordinary that when she prepares a meal she easily digests all three worlds. Greed lives by serving her.

---

144. *Jnaneshwari*, III, 225-233.
145. *Bhagavad Gita*, III, 37.

"Infatuation highly honors desire and anger. Ego, too, does business with them, and this is why it makes the world dance for its delight. Hypocrisy, which robs truth of its essence and replaces it with the straw of falsehood, also lives in their world. Desire and anger loot peace, adorn the beggar delusion, and pollute holy men. They devastate the haven of discrimination, stripping dispassion bare and twisting the neck of tranquility. They destroy the forest of contentment, demolish the fortress of courage, and up-root the plant of joy. They wreck the understanding of unity, wipe out even the name of happiness, and kindle the fire of the three afflictions in the heart of the world. When they come into contact with a person's body, they cling to him and cannot be found even by Brahma.

"They are neighbors of Consciousness and are seated alongside wisdom, and once they begin their work nothing can stop them. Silently, they seize all beings. They can drown without water and burn without fire. They kill without weapons, bind without ropes, and strike down a wise person for a wager. They bury one without earth and ensnare one without a noose. Because their strength is matchless, they are undefeated." [146]

The Mystery of Karma

People think a great deal about actions and how to become free of them; they wonder how to perform actions and yet remain detached from them. It is important to find answers to these questions. What do the *Bhagavad Gita* and *Jnaneshwari* say?

kim karma kim akarmeti kavayo'pyatra mohitāhā,
tat te karma pravakshyāmi yajjnātvā mokshyase'shubhāt. [147]

---

146. *Jnaneshwari,* III, 234-254.
147. *Bhagavad Gita,* IV, 16.

"What is action? What is inaction? This matter confuses even the wise. Therefore, I will teach you the nature of action and inaction, by knowing which you will be liberated from the evil of the wheel of birth and death."

"Even wise people become perplexed while thinking about the nature of action and inaction. Just as a counterfeit coin appears to be real and deceives the eyes, so, in the delusion of nonattachment, even men with the power to manifest another creation become involved in actions. When this is the case, what about the foolish? Pondering this question, even those wise beings who can foretell the future become deceived. For this reason, I will explain the nature of action to you very clearly. Listen."[148]

karmano hyapi boddhavyam cha vikarmanaha,
akarmanash cha boddhavyam gahana karmano gatihi.[149]

"For the true nature of action enjoined by the scriptures, as well as that of unlawful action and of inaction, should be known; the natural path of action is difficult to understand."

"Action refers to the spontaneous creation of the universe. First, thoroughly understand this natural action. Next, understand the actions that the scriptures prescribe for the different castes and stages of life, as well as their purpose. Then, completely understand the forbidden actions, and you will no longer be perplexed or confused. In reality, action is so universal that the entire world teems with it. In this context, I shall discuss only the necessary characteristics."[150]

karmanyakarma yah pasyed akarmani cha karma yaha,
sa buddhimān manushyeshu sa yuktah krutsnakarmakrut.[151]

---

148. *Jnaneshwari*, IV, 84-87.
149. *Bhagavad Gita*, IV, 17.
150. *Jnaneshwari*, IV, 88-91.
151. *Bhagavad Gita*, IV, 18.

"He who sees inaction in action and action in inaction is wise among men; he is a yogi and a performer of all actions."

"The sense of inaction has fully entered a person who, even while carrying out his duties, knows that he is action-less, who, although performing actions, has no desire for their fruits, and who acts only out of a sense of duty. One who performs all his actions regularly and properly and who possesses the above-mentioned characteristics should be considered wise.

"A man standing near water sees his own reflection in it, yet knows that he is different from the reflection. A person in a boat watches the trees on the bank passing rapidly by, yet when he ponders the matter he realizes that the trees are motionless. In the same way, a person who understands that from the viewpoint of the Self the performance of actions is illusory, and who recognizes his own original nature, truly performs no actions. Because of its rising and setting, the sun appears to move, but in reality it is motionless. In the same way, although that being performs all actions, he maintains a state of inaction. He looks like a mere human being, yet he is untouched by human nature just as the sun, although reflected in water, is not drenched by the water. Such a being perceives the universe, does everything, and enjoys all pleasures, yet remains still, completely detached from all these actions. Although seated in one place, he travels through the entire universe; in fact, it would be more accurate to say that he becomes the universe. When he attains full understanding of detachment from actions, he is not touched by the bondage of actions although he performs all actions; even after performing them, he remains the nondoer."[152]

---

152. *Jnaneshwari*, IV, 92-101.

The Importance of Knowledge

Knowledge, whether mundane or spiritual, is very important. Mundane activities cannot be carried out properly without knowledge. But in spirituality, knowledge is even more vital because the attainment of the ultimate state comes through knowledge. Knowledge eliminates all faults and sins; the fire of knowledge that blazes in meditation consumes all defects. The *Bhagavad Gita* explains its importance:

sreyān dravyamayādyajñāj jñānayajnah parantapa,
sarvam karmākhilam pārtha jñāne parisamāpyate. [153]

"Knowledge as a sacrifice is greater than any material sacrifice, O Parantapa [scourge of the foe], for all works without exception culminate in wisdom."

tadviddhi pranipātena pariprashnena sevayā,
upadekshyanti te jñānam jñāninas tattvadarsinaha. [154]

"Learn this by humble reverence, by inquiry, and by service. The men of wisdom who have seen the Truth will instruct you in knowledge."

"O Arjuna, the happiness of heaven is the highest reward of the external ceremonies and fire rituals that are mentioned in the Vedas and in which only material objects are offered in sacrifice. But just as the light of the stars fades when the sun rises, all material sacrifices seem trivial when compared to the *yajna* [fire sacrifice] of knowledge. That knowledge is like a divine lotion[155] for the eyes. Yogis who attain it feel that they have found a secret treasure of supreme joy and do not let it slip away from them. That knowledge is the final goal of current actions, the storehouse of the understanding of inaction, and the source of

---

153. *Bhagavad Gita,* IV, 33.
154. Ibid., IV, 34.
155. Which gives the vision of unity.

satisfaction for restless seekers. By attaining that knowledge, a yogi's attachment to action is weakened, his power of reason is blinded, his senses forget to contact the sense objects, his mind loses its activity, and his tongue forgets its power of speech. This knowledge fulfills his desire for renunciation, satisfies his sense of discrimination, and easily makes him attain the Self. If you wish to acquire that highest wisdom, you must serve holy men and saints with a pure mind. Service to such beings is the threshold to the temple of knowledge. Therefore, O Arjuna, attain knowledge by performing service with great enthusiasm. Prostrate at their feet with body, mind, and soul. Serve them in all humility. When you serve holy men, they will explain to you whatever you ask, and if the teaching of this knowledge penetrates your heart, all your thoughts will vanish."[156]

yajjnātvā na punarmohamevam yāsyasi pāndava,
yena bhūtānyasheshena drakshyāsyātmanyatho mayi. [157]

"Knowing That, O Pandava, you will not again become deluded like this; for by this knowledge you will see all beings in your Self and also in Me."

"By the light of that state, the mind becomes fearless and is transformed into Brahman Himself. By attaining that state, O Arjuna, you will see yourself as well as all other beings in My eternal form. O Arjuna, when you receive the Guru's grace, the morning of wisdom will dawn and the darkness of ignorance will be dispelled."[158]

api chedasi pāpebhyah sarvebhyah pāpakruttamaha,
sarvam jnānaplavenaiva vrujinam santarishyasi. [159]

---

156. *Jnaneshwari*, IV, 156-166.
157. *Bhagavad Gita*, IV, 35.
158. *Jnaneshwari*, IV, 167-169.
159. *Bhagavad Gita*, IV, 36.

"Even if you are the most sinful of all sinners, you will truly cross over all sin by the raft of knowledge."

"You may be an ocean of sins, a storehouse of ignorance, or a mountain of defects, but compared to the power of the supreme knowledge, all these things are insignificant. This knowledge has extraordinary and sublime power. If the illusory universe, which is the shadow of the formless Supreme Principle, cannot equal the light of knowledge, how much effort must this knowledge make to remove the impurities of your mind? To harbor any doubts about this is sheer madness. There is nothing in this world as great or as all-encompassing as knowledge." [160]

yathaidhāmsi samiddho'gnir bhasmasāt kurute'rjuna,
jnānāgnih sarvakarmāni bhasmasāt kurute tathā. [161]

"As a blazing fire reduces fuel to ashes, O Arjuna, so does the fire of knowledge reduce all actions to ashes."

"At the time of the final dissolution, all three worlds will burn and disperse into space like smoke. How could ordinary clouds withstand such destruction? If the fire of the final dissolution, aided by the power of the wind, will burn even water, how can it be suppressed by grass and sticks?" [162]

na hi jnānena sadrusham pavitramihi vidyate,
tat svayam yogasamsiddhah kālenātmani vindati. [163]

"There is nothing on earth equal in purity to wisdom. In the course of time, he who is perfected in yoga finds himself in the Self."

---

160. *Jnaneshwari,* IV, 170-173.
161. *Bhagavad Gita,* IV, 37.
162. *Jnaneshwari,* IV, 174-175.
163. *Bhagavad Gita,* IV, 38.

"If you think about it carefully, you find that it is incorrect to say that the impurity of the mind cannot be removed by supreme knowledge. There is nothing purer than knowledge. Just as in the world there is nothing but Consciousness and nothing that can be compared to it, this knowledge is so sublime that nothing can equal it. If there were another heavenly body as brilliant as the sun, if the sky could be tied in a bundle, or if you could lift the weight of the whole earth in your hand, only then, O Arjuna, could you find something in this world comparable to that knowledge. Therefore, examined from every point of view and considered again and again, it becomes certain that the purity of knowledge can be found only in knowledge and nowhere else. The taste of nectar can be described only as nectarean, and in the same way knowledge can be compared only to knowledge."

When Shri Krishna said this, Arjuna replied, "O Lord, what You say is true." Then he thought, "I should ask Shri Krishna about the characteristics of this knowledge and how to recognize it."

Precisely at that moment, Shri Krishna understood Arjuna's thoughts and said, "O Arjuna, I will tell you how to acquire this knowledge."[164]

sraddhāvān labhate jñānam tatparah samyatendriyaha,
jñānam labdhvā parām sāntimachirenādhigacchati.[165]

"A man who is full of faith, who is devoted to [knowledge], and who has subdued his senses attains this knowledge. Having gained knowledge, he attains supreme peace."

"There is no doubt that one who after tasting the bliss of the Self considers all objects of sense insignificant, who does not nourish his senses, whose mind causes him no trouble, who does not forget himself in *maya*, and who

---

164. *Jnaneshwari,* IV, 176-184.
165. *Bhagavad Gita,* IV, 39.

becomes happy in the company of faith is sought out by
that knowledge, which is complete and filled with perfect
peace. When knowledge is established in the heart and
peace arises, knowledge of the Self blossoms and spreads.
Then wherever one looks one sees only peace, and one's
idea of self and others is completely destroyed. In this
way, the seed of knowledge continually and endlessly
flourishes. How much can I describe it? It is enough to say
this."[166]

The Supreme Worship

In our Ashram, Gurudev Siddha Peeth, great emphasis is
placed on chanting—the repetition of God's name—and
mantra. Chanting sessions are held regularly. All the great
Siddhas chanted, for to remember the name is to remember
the living God. The name is God in a manifest form, the
perfect Parabrahman, the sound that emanates from the
inner space of God. Only one who is well versed in the
science of sound can understand the effects of sound. Sound
is the power of the *matruka shakti*, the *shakti* that manifests
initially in the form of sound. Chanting is Brahman in the
form of sound vibrations. It is the means as well as the goal.
In the *Bhagavad Gita* it is said:

*mahātmānastu mām pārtha daivim prakrutimāshritāhā,
bhajantyananyamanaso jnātvā bhūtādimavyayam.* [167]

"The great souls, O Arjuna, who abide in My divine nature,
knowing Me as the imperishable source of all beings, worship Me with an undistracted mind."

"I, who am a *kshetra sannyasi*,[168] dwell in the hearts of
those great beings. The detachment of those beings does

---

166. *Jnaneshwari*, IV, 185-190.
167. *Bhagavad Gita*, IX, 13.
168. One who has taken a vow always to remain in the same pure place.

not leave them even during sleep. The kingdom of righteousness lies in their pure feelings of faith, and the dew of discrimination lies in their minds. They have bathed in the river of wisdom, and having attained the state of the perfect Brahman, they are content. They are like shoots issuing from Parabrahman; for them the world has come to an end. They are the cornerstones of patience and are like pitchers filled to the brim with the water of the ocean of bliss. Their spirit of devotion is so fervent that they dismiss liberation, saying, 'Stay away! We don't need you.' Morality resides in their daily activities, and peace adorns all their senses. Their minds are so expanded that they envelop My all-pervasive being. These all-powerful great beings know My true nature completely. Fortunate in possessing divine wealth, they worship Me with ever-increasing love, and the sense of separation does not touch them in the slightest. O Arjuna, they have become Me, and living in that state of oneness with Me, they naturally serve Me. Listen to the wonders which proceed from that service."[169]

satatam kīrtayanto mām yatantashcha dridhavratāhā,
namasyantashcha mām bhaktyā nityayuktā upāsate. [170]

"Always glorifying Me, striving, firm in their vows, prostrating before Me, they worship Me with devotion, always steadfast."

"In the intensity of their devotion, such devotees dance with great joy during the chanting of divine names. They have eliminated the necessity for all acts of repentance because there is no taint of sin in them. They have also eliminated the need for rules of conduct and self-control, wiped away all places of pilgrimage, and closed off the path that leads to the world of death. The rules of conduct

---

169. *Jnaneshwari,* IX, 187-195.
170. *Bhagavad Gita,* IX, 14.

ask, 'If these people have already brought the senses under their control, what is there for us to curb?' Seeing that they have mastered their minds, self-control asks, 'What is there for me to subdue?' Pilgrimage asks, 'Since there are no faults in them for my remedies to cure, what should I wash away with my purity?' While chanting My name, the great beings remove all pain from the world and fill the entire universe with the bliss of the Self. They make the day of knowledge dawn without the rising of the sun, make people deathless without the nectar of immortality, and enable them to behold liberation without practicing yoga. They do not know how to distinguish between a king and a beggar, big and small, high and low; therefore, they keep the vessel of bliss open to the whole world. Rarely does anyone reach Vaikuntha, the abode of God, but these beings make the entire universe Vaikuntha. In this way, through chanting, they purify the whole world and make it radiant. They are effulgent like the sun, yet the sun is defective because it sets. The moon, too, becomes full only at certain times, but these beings are always whole. Clouds give generously, but now and then their wealth is depleted. For that reason, they are also unable to equal these great beings. Truly, these beings should be called lions. To utter My name only once, one has to pass through thousands of lifetimes, and that name constantly dances on their tongues with great love. I do not dwell in Vaikuntha, nor am I seen in the orb of the sun. More than that, I transcend even the minds of yogis. Yet, O Arjuna, I can easily be found where devotees chant My name ardently with love.

"Just see how and to what extent these beings merge into My nature. They forget even time and place and attain the bliss of the Self while chanting My name. Their repetition of 'Krishna,' 'Vishnu,' 'Hari,' and 'Govinda' goes on incessantly. They speak of the Self with hearts completely open to Me; brimming with love, they sing of My qualities.

Enough has been said. O Arjuna, these devotees move among animate and inanimate objects while chanting My name. With great effort, they restrain their five vital airs, suppress the mind completely, and bring it under their control. Erecting a wall of control and restraint, they build within it a protective barrier of the *vajra* posture, and on these barricades they mount the cannons of breath control. Then light shines forth as a result of the awakening of the Kundalini Shakti. In that light, with the help of the mind and the vital force, the nectarean lake of perfect Self-knowledge is revealed. Then it is time for the indrawn senses to become completely one-pointed, as they reach the highest stage of concentration. The words produced by mental modifications cease to exist, and all the senses are drawn to the heart and sealed off. The horsemen of the perfect state of meditation dash about rounding up the five elements, and the four divisions of the army of thoughts and doubts are vanquished. Then the victorious battle cry resounds: 'The victory is won! The victory is won!' The drums of concentration and meditation are beaten, and unity with Brahman shines forth in its supremacy. After this, in the kingdom of Self-realization, *abhisheka* is performed to the Goddess Lakshmi in the form of the state of *samadhi*.

"O Arjuna, chanting My name is profound and mysterious. The devotees who chant My name understand that just as there is only thread running through a woven garment from one end to the other, I pervade all things, animate and inanimate. They recognize that there is no object in which I do not dwell, knowing that everything in this world shares My nature, from Brahma at the beginning to an insect at the end, along with all the beings in the middle. They see no difference between great and small, animate and inanimate; whatever object they perceive they know to be My own Self, a form of Brahman. They are even unaware of their own greatness, because they do not distinguish between the worthy and the unworthy. They like to respect all people with humility; just as rain that has fallen from above collects and then pours down as a waterfall, it is their nature to offer respect to everyone they see. Just as the branches of a tree laden with fruit naturally bend toward the ground, they unaffectedly humble themselves before all creatures. They are always free of conceit. Considering humility to be their wealth, they offer it to Me while reciting words of homage. Because they have humbled themselves before all, their sense of honor and dishonor has been destroyed. They have become one with Me and, always absorbed in Me, they worship Me.

"O Arjuna, I have described to you the true and essential devotion. Now hear about those who worship Me through the *yajna* of knowledge. O Arjuna, you already know the method of worship, for I have explained it to you."

Listening to Krishna's words, Arjuna replied, "O Lord, it is true that I have already had the good fortune of receiving that *prasad*. But if nectar is served again and again, will anyone say, 'Stop! I don't want any more'?"

Hearing Arjuna, Shri Krishna understood that he had begun to savor the subject, that his heart was swaying in the bliss of knowledge. Therefore, Shri Krishna said, "Very good, Arjuna. You have spoken well. This is really not the occasion to discuss the matter, but the love and respect that I have in My heart for you force Me to speak."

Hearing this, Arjuna said, "O Lord, what are You saying? Does not the moon send forth its rays even in the absence of the *chakora* bird? Is it not the nature of the moon to remove the heat of the world? Just as the *chakora* bird keeps its beak open out of love and stares at the moon, I also make a small request of You. But, O Lord, You are the sea of compassion. With their power, clouds quench the thirst of the world. Compared to the showers that stream from the clouds, the thirst of the *chataka* bird is very small. But to obtain even a mouthful of water, one must go to a river. In the same way, whether my request is small or great, please explain this to me in detail."

Hearing Arjuna, the Lord said, "Say no more. After the joy that I have experienced, there is no room for the praise that comes from your lips. You have been listening to Me with a true heart, which moves Me to speak more."[171]

The Mystery of the Yajna of Knowledge

The scriptures say that the supreme state can be attained through knowledge. In his commentary on the *Gita*, Jnaneshwar discusses the secret of the *yajna* of knowledge. His description is very mysterious. He states that only knowledge itself can be compared to knowledge. It is knowledge of one's own true nature that is *yajna*, not the knowledge of scriptures, philosophies, or other external things, but the pure knowledge of the Self, the ever-present experience of Consciousness that arises in a pure heart.

jnānayajnene chāpyanye yajanto māmupāsate,
ekatvena pruthaktvena bahudhā vishvatomukham. [172]

"Others again sacrifice with the sacrifice of wisdom, and worship Me as the One, the distinct, and the manifold, facing in all directions."

"Now I shall explain to you how you can acquire the *yajna* of knowledge. Parabrahman's primal thought, 'Let Me become many,' is the pillar of the *yajna*. The five elements are the canopy, and the sense of separateness is the sacrificial animal. The special qualities of the five ele-

---

171. *Jnaneshwari*, IX, 196-237.
172. *Bhagavad Gita*, IX, 15.

ments, the senses, and the vital airs are the materials used in the *yajna* of knowledge. Ignorance is the *ghee* used as the oblation, and the mind and intellect are the pits in which the fire of knowledge burns. O friend Arjuna, the balanced mind should be considered the altar. The sharpness and discrimination of the intellect are the power of the mantras, peace is the vessel, and the individual soul is the sacrificer. Reciting the great mantra of discrimination, the sacrificer offers the sense of duality to the fire of knowledge from the vessel of the experience of the Absolute. Thus, ignorance is destroyed and when, at the end of the *yajna*, the individual bathes in the water of union with the Self, both sacrificer and sacrifice cease to exist. Then he no longer regards the five elements, the senses, or the sense objects as different; when the intellect is reflected in the unity of the Self, everything becomes Brahman. O Arjuna, a man upon awakening says, 'Was it not I who while sleeping was that strange army in my dream? The dream army was part of a web of delusion, and I was and still am all that.' In the same way, a person who performs the *yajna* of knowledge understands that the entire universe is not different from Brahman. Thus, his idea that he is an individual soul is destroyed; he is filled with the knowledge of God and attains the state of Brahman.

"In this way, realizing unity, some people worship Me through the *yajna* of knowledge. There are some devotees who believe that this universe is without beginning. Everyone in the universe is one, appearing different because of the diversity of names and forms. Although for this reason there seems to be duality, there is no duality in the understanding of these devotees. The limbs appear to be separate, but they belong to the same body. Whether the branches are big or small, they are part of the same tree. Although there are countless rays of sunlight, they all belong to one sun. In the same way, all the different names, forms, activities, and the duality that corresponds to them belong to this one universe. My devotees know that I am completely free of duality. O Arjuna, those who do not allow the sense of duality to touch their awareness of Brahman perform the *yajna* of knowledge correctly. No matter when or where they look, and regardless of what they see, they understand that nothing exists except Me, Parabrahman.

"Look! Bubbles may form but they are still water, and whether they burst or float they remain in water. When the wind blows, particles of dust may fly here and there, but their identity with the earth is never destroyed, and when they fall they come to rest on the same earth. Similarly, an object is always Brahman, whatever its name or form, whether it exists or ceases to exist. Because I am all-pervasive, the devotees' experience of Brahman is also all-encompassing, and they perform their various activities while maintaining the awareness that this manifold universe is the one Brahman. O Arjuna, just as a person who wants to see the sun finds it directly before him, these beings who see the world through their awareness of Brahman see their own Self in everything. O Arjuna, there is not the slightest duality in their knowledge. Just as the wind is equally present in all quarters of the sky, their awareness equally pervades the entire universe; their knowledge of Brahman is as pervasive as I Myself. Therefore, even if they do not perform acts of worship, their worship of Me automatically takes place. In fact, since I alone exist everywhere, who does not continually worship Me? Yet, since not all these people have the all-pervasive awareness, they do not attain My real nature. It is not necessary for Me to elaborate this here. I have explained to you how I am worshipped through the *yajna* of right knowledge. Whatever actions are performed are ultimately offered to Me. But the ignorant, being unaware of this mystery, do not attain My pure nature."[173]

---

173. *Jnaneshwari*, IX, 238-263.

The Doer of Nonaction

The characteristics of those whose false ego has been destroyed, who are unaffected by actions, and who remain free of sin even after performing all actions are explained in Jnaneshwar's commentary on the eighteenth chapter of the *Bhagavad Gita*.

yasya nāhamkrito bhāvo buddhiryasya na lipyate,
hatvāpi sa imān lokān na hanti na nibadhyate. [174]

"He who is free of the sense of ego, whose intelligence is not tainted by good or evil, though he slays these people, he neither slays nor is bound by the action."

"O wise Arjuna, the individual soul has been sleeping in ignorance throughout infinity, caught up in manifold dreams. But suddenly he hears the great truth *tat tvam asi*—'Thou art That'—while the hand of the Guru's grace strikes his head. At once, he is awakened from his sleep of illusion and from his cosmic dream and becomes aware of the bliss of union with the Self. The waves that appear clearly in a mirage vanish in the moonlight. One whose childhood has come to an end is no longer afraid of a goblin. Once fuel has been burned, it cannot be used again as fuel. After awakening, one no longer sees dreams and, similarly, in such a soul ego-awareness completely vanishes. The sun could not find darkness even if it entered a tunnel or a cavern, because wherever the sun goes it floods everything with light. In the same way, when a person who is filled with the awareness of the Self looks at visible objects, then for him those objects become identical with the seer. By mingling with them, he becomes one with them. If fire comes in contact with any object, that object also becomes fire, and then the duality of that which burns and that which is burned is destroyed. In the same

---

174. *Bhagavad Gita*, XVIII, 17.

way, when actions are no longer considered to be separate from the Self, when the false imputation that the Self is the doer and originator of actions is laid to rest, whatever remains is the state of the Self. How can one who attains mastery of that state remain bound to the body? How can the boundless water of the deluge merge into a mere stream or even conceive of the independent existence of a stream? O Arjuna, how can the 'I'-consciousness, the identity with the Self of all which arises when unity becomes perfect, merge into petty identification with the body? Can the reflection of the sun suppress the sun itself? When butter, which is unattached by nature, has been churned from milk, how can it again blend with buttermilk? O Arjuna, best among the brave! Once the fire concealed in wood is removed from it, can it ever again be confined to the wood? Can the effulgent sun which emerges from the womb of night ever remain in the dark? Similarly, when a person eliminates the duality between the knower and the known, how can the petty notion 'I am the body' arise in him? Wherever space extends it is filled with space, for it is eternally all-pervasive. In the same way, when such a person sees his own Self in everything he does, for what action can he be responsible as the doer? Space has no place of its own to live, the ocean has no independent currents, and the North Star has no movement; similarly, such an individual does not perform actions.

"His sense of individuality has been burned to ashes by his awareness of the Self, yet action continues as long as his body exists. After the wind ceases to blow, the trees keep swaying for a while. The fragrance of camphor remains in a vessel even after the camphor has been consumed, and when a song is finished the trance-like state experienced by the listeners lingers. Even after water has flowed by, moisture remains in the ground for a while. After the sun has set, its light blazes like a lamp on the horizon. After an arrow is shot through a target, it continues to move until its force is spent. When a potter removes from his wheel the pot he has made, the wheel goes on revolving for a while at the same speed. In the same way, even when the sense of individuality ceases, O Arjuna, the inherent nature through which the body was created impels the body to perform actions. A dream may arise without previous thought, trees grow in a forest without having been planted, and clouds take the form of castles without having been built. In the same way, although the Self performs no actions, all actions automatically take place through the five bodily organs of action. As a result of past deeds, the five causes and the five organs perform many actions, but the Self does not wonder whether those actions destroy the entire world or create a new one any more than the sun wonders why lotuses wither or why they bloom. The earth may be split asunder by bolts of lightning, or quiet, gentle showers may cause it to bring forth grass and greenery, but the sky remains unaware of any of these things. In the same way, a liberated being who lives in the body yet is beyond body-consciousness does not notice whether bodily actions create or destroy something any more than a person who is awake dreams.

"On the other hand, those whose vision does not penetrate beyond the physical body believe that even a liberated being is entangled in actions. When a vulture sees a scarecrow that has been placed in a field to frighten away animals and birds, does it not think that the scarecrow is really guarding the field? Observers may wonder whether a madman is naked or clothed, but the madman himself is not concerned with such things. A person who dies in battle is unaware of his wounds, even though others may count them. When a devoted widow is about to immolate herself, others may wonder how she will adorn herself on her final day, but she herself is unaware of the flames, the softness of her body, or the people around her. In the same way, a being who has realized the essential nature of the Self and is no longer aware of the duality of seer and seen is unaware of the actions that his senses may perform. When the small currents of rivers merge into the vast currents of the ocean, a person standing on the shore may think that one current has swallowed another, but this is actually not the case. In the same way, for a being who has attained the state of perfection, there is no one but himself to slay. A golden statue of Chandika kills a golden statue of Mahishasura with a golden spear, and the priest who watches it considers this play to be completely real. But in truth, the Goddess Chandika, the demon Mahishasura, and the spear are all made of gold. Although fire and water are depicted in a painting, they are only a visual appearance; on the canvas itself, there is neither fire nor water. In the same way, the body of a liberated being who is beyond body-consciousness acts in accordance with the results of his past deeds, but ignorant people, failing to understand this mystery, think that he himself is the doer.

"Even if the three worlds are destroyed as a result of his inherent actions, it should never be thought that a liberated being has done this. Is it clever for a person to say, 'First I will perceive darkness with the help of light, and then I will dispel it'? Once the light appears, the darkness will vanish on its own and, similarly, in an enlightened being there is nothing other than knowledge. If nothing exists but his own Self, whom can he slay? His mind is untouched by virtue or sin, just as the Ganges is not polluted if another river merges into it. O Arjuna, if fire fights fire, which will burn which? What will happen if a weapon strikes itself? Similarly, how can actions sully the mind of a person who does not consider actions to be different from himself? Actions performed by the body cannot bind a person for whom the action, the doer of the action, and the process of performing the action have all become the Self. The individual soul, considering himself the doer, uses the ten senses as instruments and skillfully reveals the five purposes. Then building two seats—one of justice and the other of injustice—he erects in a moment a temple of actions. The Self offers no help in this great work. If you were to ask, 'Does the Self not help to plan the actions?' the answer would be that it does not even do that. Can the Self, which is witness-consciousness, ever allow itself to have any thoughts about engaging in actions? Even the agitation of the actions in which people are entangled does not touch the Self. Therefore, a being who completely becomes the Self can never be bound by actions. But when false knowledge is impressed on the screen of ignorance, then the well-known threefold concept of action, doer of action, and means of action is revealed."[175]

The Perfect Renunciant

The awareness and attainment of nonaction, the understanding of renunciation, the complete lack of desire in all actions, true understanding, and the perfect yoga of renunciation are all explained by Jnaneshwar. Considered from the correct point of view, a human being is God. Seen from the wrong point of view, the world is a mere world. Outwardly it appears to be only an object, but inwardly it is the flame of Consciousness. The *Shiva Sutras* say, *chaitanyam ātmā*[176]—"The Self is Consciousness."

asaktabuddhih sarvatra jitātmā vigataspruhaha,
naishkarmyasiddhim paramām sannyāsenādhigacchati.[177]

---

175. *Jnaneshwari*, XVIII, 392-456.
176. *Shiva Sutras*, I, 2.
177. *Bhagavad Gita*, XVIII, 49.

"By renunciation, he whose intellect is unattached every-where, who has subdued himself, and from whom desire has fled attains the supreme state of freedom from action."

"A dispassionate man cannot be bound by the body any more than the wind can be caught in a net. When fruit ripens, it cannot remain on the branch, nor can the branch hold it. Similarly, in the perfect state, one's love for worldly things is weakened. Just as no one will claim that a vessel of poison belongs to him and that only he will drink it, similarly, such a being becomes detached from his wife, children, and wealth, never regarding them as his own. He mentally detests all worldly things. His mind with-draws from all sense pleasures and enters the inner sol-itude of the heart. Even if his mind wanders outside, it has become so detached from everything that it serves him one-pointedly, like a servant who is afraid to disobey his master's command. O Arjuna, he encloses his mind with-in the grasp of unity and makes it pursue the Self. At that point, his desires for worldly and heavenly pleasures are suppressed and slain, for just as a fire is extinguished when dust and mud are thrown on it, so when the mind is controlled all its desires are destroyed. Then he attains the state of dispassion.

"O Arjuna, such a being destroys the knowledge created by illusion and becomes established in the field of true knowledge. Just as accumulated water is depleted when it is used, his past actions are destroyed as his body undergoes their consequences, and his mind does not help in any way to create new actions. O Arjuna, best among the brave! In this state of balanced *karmas*, a per-son easily finds his Sadguru. When the four watches of the night pass, the eyes automatically see the sun, the enemy of darkness. When a plantain tree bears fruit, its growth ceases, and in the same way a seeker who has attained this state of equilibrium automatically sees his Sadguru. Then, O best among the brave, he reaches perfection by the grace of the Sadguru, just as when the moon is full all its defects are removed and it becomes perfect. Ignorance is destroyed through that grace, and not even an iota remains. When the sun rises, night and darkness are put to flight. If a pregnant woman kills an animal, the child in her womb instantly dies. Similarly, the threefold idea of action, doer of the action, and means of doing the action, which lives in the womb of ignorance, is destroyed. When ignorance is annihilated, all activity also comes to an end. In this way, renunciation reaches the root of all actions, for when the root of ignorance is destroyed, names and forms—the foundation of illusory actions—are also destroyed. Then one becomes the embodiment of knowledge. If a man dreams that he is drowning in a deep river, does he try to rescue himself after he awakens and his nightmare comes to an end? Similarly, in his dream, a man may think that he lacks understanding and may want to attain knowledge. But when he awakens, he becomes free of the ideas of knower and process of knowing; he becomes knowledge itself. O Arjuna, best among the brave! When a mirror is taken away, the reflections that were seen in it also vanish and only the seer is left. Similarly, when ignorance is destroyed, even the knower disappears and only actionless Consciousness remains. O Arjuna, because it is not the nature of Consciousness to perform actions, it is said to be beyond action.

"When the wind ceases to blow, the waves merge with the ocean and become the ocean, and in the same way, when his sense of duality, born of ignorance, is destroyed, a person attains his original nature. Then the sense of nonaction and the destruction of differences arise. The attainment of nonaction is the most significant and sublime of all attainments. The dome is the pinnacle of a temple, a river merges into the ocean, and absolute purity gives gold its highest value. In the same way, when both knowledge and ignorance are eliminated and one reaches this state, nothing else remains to be done. Therefore, it is called the supreme attainment."[178]

The Characteristics of One Who Has Attained Brahman

Jnaneshwar describes the characteristics of a being who has become free of misery and desire and who, because he has perceived God, considers all beings to be equal.

brahmabhūtah prasannātmā na shochati na kānkshati,
samah sarveshu bhūteshu madbhaktim labhate parām.[179]

"Becoming Brahman, serene in the Self, he neither grieves nor desires; regarding all beings as alike, he obtains supreme devotion to Me."

"O Arjuna, when a person becomes worthy of uniting with Brahman, he becomes settled in the seat of mental contentment, which results from the wisdom of Brahman. Food that has been cooked can be eaten with enjoyment after it cools off. The turbulent floods of a river subside after the rainy season, and at the end of a song the accompanying drum beat dies out. In the same way, all the stress of striving after Self-realization vanishes the moment one attains it. This serene and joyful state is called the glory of Self-realization. In it one is flooded with the awareness of one's unity with Brahman. A person in this state does not suffer if he loses something, nor does he strive to attain anything; he is subject to neither the pain of loss nor the desire for gain. Just as when the sun rises all the stars lose their brilliance, so everything else fades

---

178. *Jnaneshwari*, XVIII, 947-972.
179. *Bhagavad Gita*, XVIII, 54.

when he experiences the nature of the Self. O Arjuna, no matter where such a person may look, the diverse creation of countless beings no longer exists for him. Just as letters written on dust can be wiped away with the hand, so all forms of disparity disappear from his view. The false knowledge that arises in both the waking and dream states merges into primordial ignorance, and as the knowledge of Brahman increases, ignorance also passes away, ultimately merging into perfect wisdom. When a person eats, his hunger decreases with every morsel of food, and when he becomes completely satisfied, his hunger is entirely eliminated. As one walks along a road, the distance to one's destination grows shorter and finally the road ends. As the waking consciousness becomes active, sleep is overcome, and when one is wide awake, sleep completely vanishes. When the moon is full, the waxing phase ceases and the bright half of the month comes to an end. In the same way, by eliminating the existence of all known objects, both knower and knowledge merge into Me, and then ignorance finally disappears. At the time of the final deluge, the forms of rivers and oceans are annihilated and the entire cosmos is filled with water. When all pots and houses are destroyed, only indivisible space exists equally everywhere. When wood is burned up, only fire is left. When ornaments fall into a jeweler's melting pot, their forms are destroyed and the gold has no name, form, or separate existence. When a man awakens and his dreams vanish, he alone exists. When a being does not see or recognize anyone but Me— not even himself—he has reached the fourth state of devotion.

"There are three paths followed by the three kinds of devotees, the afflicted, the seekers of knowledge, and those who desire wealth. But these are different from the fourth state of devotion. I call this *jnana bhakti* or the fourth state of devotion, yet it is neither one of these three nor the fourth, neither the first nor the last. This devotion is the natural state of My own being.

"O Arjuna, My inherent light destroys the darkness of ignorance which creates perplexity regarding Me. Through its help, people can easily see My nature. It engages people in worship of Me and grants them true knowledge. The miracle of this light is that wherever a person who has faith may sit, it allows him to see everything. Through this light, the universe comes into being and is dissolved, just as both dreaming and not dreaming depend on one's existence. This light is called devotion. In an afflicted person, devotion takes the form of pain. My devotee thinks of Me as that which will remove his pain; he makes Me the object of his longing, and through this form of devotion his pain is removed. O Arjuna, best among the brave, to one who seeks knowledge, devotion reveals itself as a desire for knowledge. That devotee considers Me the object of his search for knowledge, and I become that for him. In one who seeks wealth, devotion becomes the desire for wealth, O Arjuna. By identifying Me with wealth, his devotion gives Me that form. In this way, when devotion springs from ignorance, it makes a person feel that I, the seer, am that which is seen. There is no doubt that [in a mirror] the face sees the face, but it is the mirror that gives the false impression of duality. A person perceives the moon with his eyes, but if he has an eye disorder he may see two moons when there is only one. In the same way, devotees find Me everywhere through devotion, but if they think that I am the object of seeing, that is the result of their ignorance. When ignorance is dispelled, My apparent visibility and Myself become one, just as a reflection is united with the object reflected. Even when some alloy is mixed with gold, the gold itself is pure, and when the impurity is removed, only pure gold remains. Similarly, I alone exist for one who truly sees. Is not the moon complete in itself even before the night of the full moon? Of course it is, yet it seems to reach perfection on that night. In the same way, I alone am seen through the path of knowledge, although by different means, and when the seer's seeing is completely destroyed, I alone attain Myself. O Arjuna, for this reason I have said that the fourth state of devotion transcends the idea of My visibility." [180]

The Supreme Experience

Through total love, a person is absorbed into the Supreme Principle. Jnaneshwar describes the experience of all-encompassing perfection that comes to such a person as a result of knowing the Supreme Principle and attaining the outlook of Parabrahman.

bhaktyā māmabhijānāti yāvānyashchāsmi tattvataha,
tato mām tattvato jnātvā vishate tadanantaram. [181]

"By devotion he truly knows Me, what and who I am; then, having true knowledge of Me, he immediately becomes absorbed into the Supreme."

"You have already heard that the devotee, through devotion and knowledge, automatically merges into Me and that such a one is not a mere devotee but Me. O Arjuna, in the seventh chapter, I told you with authority that a wise man is My own Self. O Arjuna, at the beginning of the world, I taught this to Brahma the creator through the *Bhagavatam*. The wise call it Self-knowledge. The Shaivites call it Shakti. But I call it the highest devotion. When karma yogis become one with Me, they attain this fruit. For such a karma yogi, the world is entirely

---

180. *Jnaneshwari*, XVIII, 1106-1123.
181. *Bhagavad Gita*, XVIII, 55.

pervaded by Me. In this state, discrimination, dispassion, liberation, bondage, renunciation, and the tendencies are all destroyed. Everything comes to Me; nothing remains on the other side. All four elements—earth, water, fire, and air—are swallowed up by ether and only ether remains. Likewise, beyond the boundary that separates the goal from the means of reaching it, I, the pure and faultless Principle, alone exist. Such a being merges into that Principle, becomes one with it, and experiences the bliss of the Self.

"Remember that just as the Ganges sparkles when it merges into the ocean, he who experiences the bliss of the Self becomes that bliss. When two polished mirrors are placed in front of one another, there is beauty in their mutual reflection. In the same way, when a devotee merges into Me and becomes one with Me, he experiences the bliss of the Self. If the mirror in front of a person is removed and he can no longer see the reflection of his face, he still remains joyful within himself. A dream vanishes when one awakes, but then one enjoys one's own individual unity without the need of another. Some people say that when a person becomes one with an object, he no longer experiences that object, but one might as well ask, 'How can words utter words?' Do the people who say such things have to kindle a lamp to see the sun or build a canopy to support the sky? Can darkness ever embrace the sun? How can nonspace understand the nature of space? Can the possessor of trinkets be so proud as to consider them real jewels? In the same way, how can I exist for a person who has not become one with Me? It is unnecessary to say that he will or will not experience Me.

"Therefore, I say that a karma yogi experiences Me by becoming Me, just as a young person experiences his youth, as waves kiss the water, as light rejoices in the sun, and as space pervades the sky. When a karma yogi sees Me, he experiences Me without doing anything, just as gold ornaments experience their innate gold. Fragrance exists in sandalwood without its having to make any effort, moonlight naturally delights in the moon, and in the same way, although there is no room for action in unity, still there is a place for devotion. This cannot be described in words; it can be known only through direct experience. Whatever such a person may say about Me, because of his past merits it becomes devotion to Me, and I respond to him instantly. Then I Myself become the speaker, and when the speaker meets his own Self he cannot say anything. In that state, he can experience Me only by remaining silent. As soon as that devotee begins to speak, know that it is I who speaks through him; thus, silence bears fruit, and through silence he truly praises Me. Similarly, O Arjuna, no matter what he sees through his eyes or perceives through his mind, he perceives nothing but his own Self. Just as one who looks in a mirror sees a form that existed even before he looked in the mirror, that devotee's perception grants him the vision of his own Self. When the object that is seen disappears, the seer experiences himself as the seer, and since the act of seeing also vanishes nothing but the seer remains.

"In a dream, a wife runs to embrace a husband, but the moment she awakens she realizes that neither was he her husband nor was she his wife and, knowing this, becomes quiet. When two sticks are rubbed together, fire is produced, and then both sticks are consumed in the fire and take on its form. If the sun tries to grasp its reflection in water, the reflection will vanish and the sun, not being in its proper place, will also lose its power of being reflected. In the same way, by becoming one with Me, the devotee absorbs the object he sees into himself, and his ability to see disappears along with the object. When the sun illumines darkness, no darkness remains to be illumined, and in the same way, once the seer attains My own Self, the object to be seen is no longer visible. This state, in which there is neither visibility nor invisibility, is called true perception. O Arjuna, perceiving the same thing in whatever one sees, one experiences that vision which is beyond the duality of the seer and the seen.

"Just as space is always motionless because it pervades all space, he who has entered the nature of the Self does not move from his own place. At the time of the deluge, water alone is everywhere; since water has filled everything, there are no outflowing streams. In the same way, when the Self is full of itself, it becomes serene. How can a person step over his feet, or fire burn itself, or water give itself a bath? In the same way, when a devotee becomes wholly Me, his coming and going ceases, and then he is on the pilgrimage to union with Me. A wave on the surface of water cannot cross the land no matter how high it may leap, for the movement that impels the wave arises and subsides in water. O Arjuna, no matter how high the tide may rise, its nature as water never changes; the oneness of the waves with water is never destroyed. In the same way, when such a devotee has become wholly united with Me, he will always be My faithful pilgrim even though he may be assailed by the sense of individuality.

"If, because of the nature of his body, he performs some action, I meet him through that very action. In this state, O Arjuna, the doer and the action vanish completely, and seeing Me as his own Self, he becomes Me. If a mirror is placed before another mirror, it cannot be said to see the mirror. One cannot gild gold, nor can a lamp give light to another lamp. In the same way, because I am action, for Me to perform action could not be termed acting. Therefore, if a devotee who is one with Me performs an action, it cannot be said that he is doing it, and since he is not responsible for any action, it is the same as if he had not done it. After he has become one with Me, the fruit of whatever action he performs is nonaction. This is true devotion to Me. O Arjuna, all the actions that he performs become nonaction, and such a person serves Me through this highest worship. Whatever he says is praise of Me. In whatever he sees, there is the vision of Me, and his every movement is a step toward union with Me. Whatever he does is worship of Me, whatever he thinks is the repetition of My name, and, O Arjuna, his stillness is absorption in Me. Just as gold ornaments are one with gold, through his devotion he is always united with Me. Waves are one with water, fragrance is inherent in camphor, and the luster of a jewel is inseparable from it. Cloth is one with its threads, and a clay pot is one with clay. Likewise, a devotee remains one with Me.

"Through his one-pointed devotion and awareness of the Self, he sees Me, the seer, in all visible things. Through the three modes of consciousness—the waking, dream, and deep sleep states—and the existence of the field and the knower of the field, the entire universe, which is observed either in a manifest or in an unmanifest state, is recognized as Me, the seer. In the field of this realization, the doll of the experience of the Self begins to dance. A rope may be mistaken for a snake, but when clearly seen it is recognized as a rope. When ornaments are melted down, one realizes that they are not separate from gold. When a person understands that a wave is nothing but water, he does not consider the form of the wave to be real. If after waking one tries to measure the content of one's dream, one discovers that there is nothing apart from oneself. In the same way, a person understands, 'I am the knower in the form of all known objects, in both that which exists and that which does not exist.' He experiences everything in this way and understands, 'I am unborn and immortal; I am indestructible and imperishable; I am unprecedented and limitless joy. I am immutable, infallible, and eternal. I am the One without a second, the origin of all, both with and without form. I am the ruler as well as the ruled. I am without beginning, deathless, and fearless. I am the support as well as that which is supported. I am the all-powerful One. I am eternal and self-born. I pervade all forms. I am the inner Self of all and transcend all. I am the ancient and the new. I am nothingness as well as fullness. I am both big and small. I am all that is. I am free of activity and without duality, attachment, or grief. I am the Lord who pervades and who is pervaded. I am beyond sound, hearing, form, and race. I pervade everywhere equally. I am independent. I am the Supreme Absolute.'

"In this way, through his single-minded devotion, he truly understands Me, and what is more, he understands that the knowledge of the experience of the Self is also Me. When a man awakens from sleep, there are no more dreams, and he realizes that only he, the dreamer, exists. The sun is both the revealer as well as the revealed; they are not different. In the same way, when the objects of knowledge disappear, only the knower is left. When a person understands this, he becomes his own Self, O Arjuna, and realizes that the knowledge through which he recognizes unity is also Me, the all-powerful One. Then he knows, 'I am the Self, which is beyond both duality and unity and is the One without a second.'

"After a person awakens in this way, his idea of individuality is destroyed. When one perceives that ornaments are made of gold, they are reduced to gold. When salt dissolves into water its saltiness remains, but when the water dries up the salt loses its existence. In the same way, when a person has the awareness 'I am that Parabrahman,' he merges into the serene state of the experience of bliss. In that state, there is no more room for ideas such as 'He' and 'I'; these notions are destroyed. When camphor is burning it can be called fire, but when both the camphor and the fire disappear only space remains. When one is subtracted from one, zero remains. Similarly, when being and nonbeing dissolve, whatever is left is Me. At that point, even such words as Brahman, the

Self, and God act as obstacles to the bliss of the Self. In that state, one cannot even say, 'Nothing exists.' Then, when everything is negated, when no word is uttered, and when there is not even any understanding of knowledge and ignorance, That can be known. In this state of union, knowledge is known through knowledge, bliss is embraced through bliss, and joy is experienced through joy. Profit is gained by profit, light is embraced by light, and wonder is lost in wonder. In this state, right conduct attains peace, rest finds rest, and experience delights in experience. By planting the beautiful vine of the yoga of action, a being reaps the fruit of the immaculate Self. O Arjuna, on the royal crown of karma yoga, I am the jewel of pure Consciousness, and that being also becomes a jewel in My crown. He is the space that surrounds the dome of liberation on the temple of karma yoga.

"In the forest of this earthly existence, the yoga of action is the royal path leading to the city of union with Me. In the waters of devotion to knowledge, the current of karma yoga flows swiftly and merges into the blissful ocean of that union. O wise Arjuna, the yoga of action is so sublime that I constantly expound it to you. You cannot attain Me merely by doing *sadhana* in the right place, at the right time, and with the right objects; I exist in all, independently, in My fullness. Therefore, one need not put forth great effort to attain Me; I am attained through this yoga of action.

"It is universally accepted that the path to union with Me is known through the relationship between disciple and Guru. O Arjuna, treasures lie in the womb of the earth. Fire is latent in wood; milk is contained in the udder of a cow. But one must use some means to obtain these things. Similarly, although I am already attained, I am reached through a method.

"At this point someone may ask, 'After discussing the fruit for so long, why does Lord Krishna introduce the means?' The answer is this: The great significance of the

Bhagavad Gita is that it discusses the direct attainment of liberation from all viewpoints. Many other scriptures have explained different means to liberation, but it cannot be said that they have done so with authority. The wind can drive the clouds from the sky, but it cannot create a sun. One's hand can remove the scum from the surface of the water, but it cannot create water. In the same way, although the scriptures may remove the impurity of ignorance obstructing the vision of Self-realization, I always remain pure and am ever-revealed. All other scriptures are capable of washing away the impurity of ignorance, but they have no independent power to bring about Self-realization, and when the time comes to prove their validity, they turn to the *Gita*. When the sun illumines the east, all directions are aglow with light. In the same way, the *Bhagavad Gita* leads all the scriptures along the right path, and all scriptures receive support from it."[182] .

Devotion to the Guru

Now begins a section on devotion to the Guru. What feelings for the Guru arise in the mind of a true disciple? What is his state of mind? A phrase in the *Bhagavad Gita* describes one of the characteristics of wisdom as *acharyopasanam*, service to the Guru. Devotion to the Guru is a mysterious science. Identification with the Guru makes one a Guru. Guru, Self, and God are one and the same, and therefore love for the Guru is love for the Self. To repeat the Guru's name is to repeat the name of the Self; love for the Guru becomes love for God. God's power of grace dwells in the Guru. An individual is not the Guru; Shakti is the Guru, and that Shakti resides in one who is a Guru. Jnaneshwar Maha-

---

182. *Jnaneshwari,* XVIII, 1124-1229.

raj comments on this mystery of devotion to the Guru. Simply by reading his commentary, one experiences the awakening of an inner pulsation. The commentary occurs in the middle of Jnaneshwar's explanation of the qualities of a wise person.

amānitvam adambhitvam ahimsā kshāntirārjavam,
āchāryōpāsanam shaucham shairyamātmavinigrahaha.[183]

"Humility, unpretentiousness, noninjury, forgiveness, uprightness, service to the teacher, purity, steadfastness, and self-control."

The Lord said, "O brother Arjuna, your eye has been opened by the lotion of knowledge. Now become more vigilant, and I will grant you the understanding of true knowledge. Know that a person in whom forgiveness resides and in whom there is not the slightest trace of sadness has attained wisdom. In deep lakes there are lotuses, and in the houses of fortunate people there is wealth. In the same way, O Arjuna, a true man of knowledge is full of forgiveness."[184]

Forgiveness

"Now I will explain to you very clearly the characteristics by which you can recognize forgiveness. Listen. If a person likes ornaments, he wears them on his body with great pleasure. In the same way, a being who is full of forgiveness bears everything joyfully. Even if a mountain of the three kinds of afflictions falls on him, he does not become the slightest bit perturbed. He accepts with respect the bad as well as the good, bears honor and dishonor equally, and considers pain and pleasure to be one. He is moved by neither praise nor blame. He does not burn with heat, nor does he shiver with cold. No matter

---

183. *Bhagavad Gita*, XIII, 7.
184. *Jnaneshwari*, XIII, 338-340.

what difficulties he has to face, he neither is frightened by them nor runs away from them. Mount Meru does not feel the weight of its peak, the third incarnation of Narayan, the boar, did not feel the weight of the earth, and the earth is not oppressed by the weight of infinite beings. In the same way, such a being is not a bit frightened when the pairs of opposites attack his body. Just as the ocean, which is a storehouse of limitless water, swells its stomach to contain the water of many rivers, there is nothing which that person cannot bear and he is not even aware of that which he has tolerated. He accepts whatever befalls him, considering it a form of the Self and finding no reason to be proud of his patience. O friend Arjuna, understand that a person who practices this nondual forgiveness adds to the greatness of wisdom. O Arjuna, such a person is the support of knowledge." [185]

Uprightness

"Now I shall explain uprightness. Just as the vital force shows the same attitude of benevolence toward all, uprightness makes a person regard others without a sense of duality. Just as the sun does not shed its light on a person because it likes him and as space equally pervades everywhere, the mind of an upright person does not regard various people differently, and his behavior is the same with all. Such a person is familiar with the entire world, and he knows very well that he has had a longstanding and intimate relationship with it. Therefore, he has no idea of 'self' and 'other.' He meets everyone just as water mixes with everything and harbors no bad thoughts about anyone. His thoughts flow as easily as the wind, and no doubt or feeling touches him. Just as a child does not hesitate to go to his mother, so this being freely expresses his thoughts to others. O Arjuna, just as once the lotus has

---

185. Ibid., 341-352.

fully bloomed no petal remains closed, his mind, too, remains open, concealing nothing. Just as rays of light fall on a polished jewel, so his mind is very pure, and all the activities that take place in his mind are also clean. He never has to wonder whether or not he should say something for, not knowing how to conceal anything in his mind, he fully reveals his true experience. In his outlook, there is not the slightest bit of deception. There is no hypocrisy in his speech, nor is it unclear. He does not belittle others. All his ten senses are pure, simple, and free of treachery. Day in and day out, the gates of his five vital airs remain open, and his heart is as simple as a stream of nectar. If you see these characteristics in a person, O Arjuna, best among the brave, understand that he is the image of uprightness and that knowledge resides in him."[186]

Service to the Guru

"O wise Arjuna, now I shall explain to you the nature of devotion to the Guru. Service to the Guru is the mother of prosperity, for it makes even a distressed person attain the nature of Brahman. I want to explain devotion to the Guru very clearly to you, so pay close attention. Just as a river with all the wealth of its waters enters the ocean, just as the wisdom of the Vedas together with all the great doctrines becomes established in Brahman, just as a devoted wife surrenders all her five vital airs as well as her good and bad qualities to her beloved husband, he who offers everything to his Guru becomes the birthplace of devotion to the Guru.

"Just as a wife parted from her husband constantly thinks of him, such a devotee always remembers his Guru's house. He runs to welcome the breeze that blows

---

186. Ibid., 353-367.

from his Guru's house, then stands before it and rolls on
the ground, beseeching it to enter his own home. Carried
away by true love, he likes to direct his speech only toward
the Guru's house, for that is where his mind resides. He
lives away from the Guru in his own home only to obey
the Guru's command, just as a calf tied with a rope lies in
the cowshed. Like the calf, he continually wonders,
'When will this rope break? When and how will I see
Gurudev?' Every moment of separation from the Guru
seems longer than an age. If anyone comes to him from his
Guru's house or brings a message from the Guru, he
experiences the joy of a dead person brought back to life.
The mention of his Guru's house fills him with the elixir of
joy, like dry sprouts that are showered with nectar, like a
small fish from a pond that finds itself in the ocean, like a
destitute person who sees a hidden treasure, a blind man
who recovers his sight, or a beggar who is raised to the
throne of Indra. Upon hearing mention of his Guru's
house, he expands so much that he can easily embrace the
sky. When you see a person who has this kind of love for
his Guru's house, O Arjuna, know that the wisdom of
service always dwells in him.

"Through the force of his love, such a disciple establishes the image of his Guru in his heart, and through
meditation he worships him. In his pure heart, he makes a
temple for his Guru and firmly establishes him there.
Through his devotion, he himself becomes the Guru's
family. In the courtyard of his knowledge, within the
temple of the bliss of the Self, he installs the image of his
Guru and pours over it the nectar of meditation. When the
sun of the awareness of Brahman dawns, he fills the
basket of his intelligence with pure feeling and offers the
flowers of his feeling to Shankar in the form of his Guru.
At all three times appointed for worship—morning, afternoon, and evening—he burns the frankincense of individuality and waves the light of knowledge to his Guru.
He always offers to him the food of union with Brahman.

In this way, he becomes the worshipper and makes his Guru the object of worship. Sometimes his mind, reclining on the bed of individuality, thinks of the Guru as the husband and enjoys the bliss of his company and love. Sometimes his heart overflows with love, which he calls the ocean of milk. In the ocean of love, in the bliss of meditation, Narayan in the form of the Guru sleeps on the water in the pure bed of the cobra Shesha. He becomes Lakshmi, massaging the legs of Narayan in the form of the Guru, or he may become Garuda, standing with folded hands next to Narayan. He pictures himself as Brahma, being born from the navel of Narayan in the form of the Guru. In this way, through his love for his Guru's form, he mentally experiences the bliss of meditation. Sometimes the disciple imagines that his Guru is his mother and he is lying in her lap while being fed, and in these fantasies he experiences bliss. O Arjuna, he may think of his Guru as a mother cow standing in the cool shade of the tree of knowledge and picture himself as her calf. Sometimes he considers the Guru's grace to be water and himself to be a fish, or he feels that the Guru's grace is rain and he a plant that springs up after the showers. There is no end to the ways of love. Sometimes he imagines that he is a fledgling bird and the Guru the mother bird feeding him with her beak. Sometimes he pictures the Guru as a boat to which he is clinging for support. When the ocean is at high tide, wave after wave arises, and similarly the waves of love continually intensify his meditation. In this way, he always savors the Guru's image in his mind.

"Now I shall tell you how this disciple serves the Guru. He always feels, 'I will serve my Guru so well that he will become pleased with me and tell me to ask him for a boon.' He thinks that when the Guru truly becomes pleased, he will humbly ask him, 'O Master, I want to become all your servants and all the things you need,' and that when he requests this boon from his Master, the Guru will say, 'So be it.'

"He thinks, 'I will become all his servants. When I become all of my Guru's instruments, I will be able to experience the wonder of service to the Guru. Although the Guru is the mother of all, I will put such pressure on him through my service that he will be my mother alone. I will draw his love so strongly that he will be like a husband devoted to only one wife; in this way, I will make him take the vow of remaining in only one place, and the Guru's love will always remain in my territory. Just as the wind can never pass beyond the limits of the four quarters, I will become a cage to ensnare all of my Guru's grace. I will adorn the lady of service to the Guru with all the ornaments of my virtues. I will become a mantle of devotion covering the Guru and will allow no one else to do this. I will become the earth on which the Guru showers his blessings.'

"In this way, the disciple forms many desires in his mind. He says, 'I will become the Guru's house. I will be his servant and do all his work. I will be the threshold of the door over which my generous Guru will pass when entering or leaving his house, and I will also be his doorkeeper. I will become his shoes and will also put them on his feet. I will become his umbrella as well as the one who holds it. I will go before him to point out where the earth is high and where it is low. I will be the one who holds his hands, as well as the one who holds his flywhisk. I will become his water pitcher and will also wash his face. When he gargles, I will be the receptacle. I will become his betelnut and will also receive whatever he spits. I will make the preparations for his bath. I will become the seat on which he rests, his garments, ornaments, sandalwood paste, and all other articles for his use. I will be his cook, will serve his food, and will myself perform the *arati*. When the Guru takes his meal I will be his companion, and when the meal is over I will come forward to offer him his betelnut roll. I will remove the dishes, make his bed, and massage his legs. I will become his throne as well as his bed. When the Guru sits on the bed, I will know that my service to him has reached its culmination. I will become the fascinating subjects and entertainment that delight my Guru's mind. I will become everything that my Guru needs. When he listens to the scriptures, I will be the groups of words. When the Guru scratches his body, I will become the sensation of touch. I will become whatever object the Guru looks at with love, whatever taste his tongue savors, and whatever fragrance pleases his nose.'

"In this way, with respect to external service to the Guru, the disciple tells his mind that he will become everything that his Guru needs and that he alone will perform all service to him. As long as his body lives, he will perform this kind of service, and when he leaves his body a different kind of service to the Guru will take shape in his mind. He says, 'When I die, I will mix the earth element of my body with the earth on which the feet of my Guru walk. I will mix the watery element of my body with the water that my Guru touches. The fiery element of my body will merge with the flames of the lamp that lights my Guru's house or with the flame that he waves in *arati*. I will place my vital force by my Guru's fan, so I will have the fortune both of serving him and of touching his body. I will merge the etheric element of my body into the space where my Guru's form may be. Alive or dead, I will never stop serving my Guru, nor let anyone else serve him even for a moment; for millions of ages I will serve him.'

"A disciple has this kind of courage. His service has no limitations of time and space. When he is serving, he does not think about day or night, nor does he regard any service as either greater or less. The harder the work the Guru gives him, the fresher and stronger he becomes. Even though the work given him by the Guru may be greater than the sky, he completes it by himself. The moment he receives the Guru's command to perform any job, his body outruns his mind, competing with it to finish the work quickly. Even if the Guru is merely joking, he will sacrifice his entire life to fulfill his command. His body becomes emaciated by this service to the Guru, but he is nourished by his love for the Guru and is the abode of the Guru's command. He considers himself to be pure by virtue of the nobility of the Guru's family, regards goodness as kind behavior toward his Guru-brothers, and is addicted only to serving his Guru. He regards as his daily duties those things that belong to his Guru's religious tradition, and devoting himself to the Guru is his daily work. He regards the Guru as his deity, mother, and father and knows no other path than service to him. The Guru's door is the Truth; it is everything for him. He behaves lovingly toward his Guru's servants and relatives. The mantra of the Guru's name is always on his tongue. He pays no attention to any scriptures other than the words of his Guru. He considers the water of the Guru's feet to be superior to all the holy places in the three worlds. To find the leftovers of his Guru's meal is more important to him than the bliss of *samadhi*. O Arjuna, he is more eager to take a speck of the dust raised by the Guru's feet than he is for the joy of liberation. He alone is a true servant and disciple of the Guru. How much more can I say? Truly, there is no limit to devotion to the Guru. Because the opportunity arose, I had to explain this in so much detail; it has been too lengthy. O Arjuna, a person who has love and longing for this kind of devotion and who enjoys nothing but serving the Guru is the real cornerstone of the knowledge of the Truth. Because of him, knowledge exists. Such an enlightened devotee is God Himself; knowledge keeps all its doors open to him. Even if the entire world were filled with his knowledge, he has so much that some would be left over."

Jnaneshwar says, "O listeners, in my heart there is great longing for this kind of service to the Guru; this is why I have explained it in such great detail. Otherwise [if I am not occupied in serving him], I am maimed even though I have hands, while with regard to worship I am blind. Even when serving the Guru, I am lamer than the lame. I am mute in praising his glory, an idler who eats others' food. But one thing is certain: I have true love for my Guru in my heart, and this is what has compelled me to become involved in this long explanation. I, Jnanadeva, ask you to bear with me whatever I may say and give me an opportunity to serve you. Now I will continue this exposition in a better way."[187]

Purity

Listen. Shri Krishna, who was the incarnation of Narayan and the bearer of the weight of the earth, spoke as Arjuna listened.

Shri Krishna said, "O Arjuna, listen. The body and mind of a pure person are as pure as camphor. He is as clear as a jewel and as clean and radiant as the sun within and without. His good actions make his body clean, while inwardly he is enlightened by his wisdom; thus he is full of purity. Externally, the body is cleansed through the uttering of Vedic mantras and the application of earth and water. The power of the intellect is cleansed by service, just as sand cleans a mirror or as a stain on cloth is removed by the washerman's soap. An enlightened being is both outwardly and inwardly pure because the light of knowledge blazes within him. Otherwise, O Arjuna, if the heart is not pure, the display of outer actions serves only to deceive others. It would be like adorning a dead body, bathing a donkey in a holy river, sprinkling a bitter pumpkin with sugar, hanging flags on a deserted and broken-down house, pasting food on the body of a starving man, putting *kum-kum* on a widow, laying gold over an empty dome, or painting fruit made of clay. Showy rituals are like this, for an imitation has little value. A pitcher of wine

---

187. Ibid., 368-458.

cannot be purified by being washed in the Ganges. There-fore, knowledge should first enter the heart, and then outer cleanliness will naturally follow. Has anyone ever attained knowledge merely by performing external ac-tions and purificatory rituals? For a person who has be-come completely pure outwardly because of his good actions and whose heart has become immaculate through wisdom, the distinction between outside and inside van-ishes, and he finds the same purity everywhere. He is so faultless within that the pure feelings of his heart are revealed through his senses, just as a flame enclosed in glass sheds its light outside. Even if he sees, hears, or encounters things that give rise to doubts and useless thoughts or sow bad actions, they do not affect his mind any more than the sky is tainted by the color of the clouds. Although his senses may enjoy sense objects, he is not the slightest bit contaminated by passion, for he remains com-pletely detached from objects of sense.

"A woman embraces both her husband and her son, yet in her love for her son there is no passion. In the same way, good and evil thoughts never seep into a pure-hearted person; he knows which actions are right and which are wrong. Just as water cannot penetrate a dia-mond and pebbles cannot be cooked in boiling water, his state of mind cannot be contaminated by any thoughts. O Arjuna, this state is known as purity, and you should know that wisdom dwells here."[188]

Steadfastness

"A person in whom steadfastness resides is the life of wisdom. His body may perform actions on its own, but the equanimity of his mind is never disturbed. A cow does not lose its affection for its calf even when it wanders in a forest. A devout wife does not run after sense pleasures. The heart of a miser remains with his buried treasure no

---

188. Ibid., 460-482.

matter how far he may go from it. Similarly, the mind of a steadfast person is not disturbed by the activity of the body. The sky does not move with the fleeting clouds, the North Pole does not shift along with the movement of the stars, and when travelers walk, the road itself does not move, nor do the trees leave their places. In the same way, even while his body is being activated by the five elements, the mind of a pure person is not disturbed by any of them. Just as the earth is not moved by the force of a storm, likewise, such a person is not disturbed by extremes of pain or pleasure. He is not distressed by the misery of poverty; he neither shivers with fear and sorrow, nor dreads the death of the body. His simple mind is not swayed by hope, desire, or disease. Not even a hair of his body is disturbed when he is assaulted by contempt and dishonor or overcome by passion or desire. Even though the sky may fall on him or the earth break open, his mind remains unshaken. Just as an elephant does not run here and there if it is beaten with flowers, likewise, he is not moved by the arrows of harsh words. Mount Mandara did not bow before the waves of the milky ocean when it was being churned. The sky is not consumed by a forest fire. Similarly, no matter how many waves of pain or pleasure arise, his mind remains unaffected. Even if the world comes to an end, his courage is maintained through its own power. This state of mind is called steadfastness, O Arjuna, and one whose body and mind acquire this kind of stability is an open treasure of wisdom.

"A phantom clings to a tree, a warrior clutches his weapons, a miser keeps his wealth within his sight, a mother clasps her child to her heart, and a bee is always greedy for honey. Similarly, O Arjuna, such a person keeps strict watch over his mind and does not allow it to stand at the threshold of the senses. He always fears that some passionate creature might hear of this child of his [the mind] or that some fiend might cast the evil eye on it, and [if that were to happen] he would lose his life. Just as a strong and arrogant husband keeps his unruly wife under control, so a pure person keeps watch over his mental tendencies. He keeps his senses subdued even when his body becomes emaciated and the time comes for the *prana* to leave it. He keeps the two guards of the *yamas* and *niyamas*, the yogic restraints and observances, alert in the castle of his body at the gateway of his mind. In the three centers—*muladhara* at the base of the spine, *manipura* at the navel, and *vishuddha* at the throat—he performs the three yogic *bandhas*, or locks—*vajra, uddyana,* and *jalandhara*—and makes his mind enter the junction of *ida* and *pingala*. He puts meditation to sleep on the couch of *samadhi*, and his mind, becoming one with Consciousness, delights in That. Know that such a person has mastered his mind and that such control of the mind is the victory of knowledge. A person whose heart and mind silently and respectfully obey his every command should be considered wisdom incarnate."[189]

The Guru's Gracious Glance

In order to explain the subject of devotion to the Guru with absolute accuracy, I have used Jnaneshwar's great devotion to his Guru as an example. The subtler the understanding with which one reads this, the more one will experience the Self of all. The passage that describes true devotion to the Guru reveals Jnaneshwar's all-pervasive awareness. Its meaning is that one must become everything, and then one's own Self will manifest in all. Many people wonder, "What sort of technique is this devotion to the Guru?" It is a highly mysterious technique, and to know it one must know the Supreme Truth. Why is devotion to the Guru so mysterious? It is said that the Guru, the Self, and God are one. That which

---

189. Ibid., 483-510.

we call the Self is God, that which we call God is the Guru, and that which we call the Guru is the Self.

Now Jnaneshwar's commentary on devotion to the Guru continues:

O gracious glance of the Sadguru! You are the grace-bestowing power. It is known to all that you are pure and sublime and shower bliss unceasingly. I bow to you. Perceiving duality is like being bitten by a snake. Your power keeps the limbs from stiffening and instantly extracts the venom. When the waves of your grace and the nectar of love begin to leap up and overflow their banks, who can be distressed, afflicted, or scorched by sorrow? O gracious and compassionate glance of the Guru! Brimming with love, you reveal to disciples the bliss of the Absolute and satisfy their yearning for Self-realization. O grace-bestowing power! You place disciples like children in the lap of Parashakti in the *muladhara chakra* at the base of the spine. Lovingly you care for them, cradling them in the space of the heart and fanning them with the knowledge of the Self. You adorn them with supreme bliss and nurse them with the elixir of perfection. You take away their idea of individuality and give them the mind and the vital airs as playthings. You sing the ten divine songs of the heart [*anahat*] to delight them, and then lull them to sleep, quieting them with the bliss of *samadhi*. Thus, you are the mother who nurtures all seekers. Knowledge, as well as the art of poetry, springs from your feet, and for that reason I will never depart from your cool shade. O gracious glance of the Sadguru! One who attains the elixir of your compassion becomes Brahma, the creator of the entire world of knowledge. O gracious glance of the Sadguru! O Mother! You are sublime. You are the wish-fulfilling tree, which grants the desires of perfect devotees. You are my mother and my father; to the wise you are everything. You are my heart. My infinite salutations to you. [190]

---

190. Ibid., XII, 1-9.

The Awareness of Oneness

It is natural for one to become that which one thinks about. If one contemplates the world with correct understanding, one will see that it is the embodiment of one's feeling. All people are the same, yet the world exists in a state of differentiation. One person says, "I am a Sufi." Another says, "I am a Moslem." A third says, "I am a Christian." Others call themselves Jews, Hindus, Vaishnavites, Buddhists, or Sikhs. The one humanity has spread out in infinite forms. If one's body is analyzed from the standpoint of Truth, it contains nothing but seven components: bones, marrow, blood, and so on. The same seven components exist in people of every race, but even though there is no fundamental difference, there are many races and religions, and people treat one another differently according to their feelings and attitudes. When truly all people are one, what is the reason for this disparity?

First, there is custom. Second, there is the sense of difference and enmity among religions; instead of developing godliness and brotherhood, people intensify their hatred toward one another. This is ignorance not only of the world, but also of the true nature of religion, and is caused chiefly by incomplete understanding of religion. When one develops correct understanding, one looks at the world with perfect vision, knowing what it really is. Then one knows the true mystery of religion. All religious people claim, "My religion is not petty. It was created by God and is superior to all others." But this is a myopic view of religion. If God had made some religions superior to others, He would have been engaging in religious politics and thus would not be God. Religious people have tainted Him with this idea; every religious person should realize that his feelings of superiority and inferiority defile God and destroy the awareness that all people belong to God's family. Such an attitude can never be true religion. Every sect creates its own holy book and uses it as a weapon to shatter universal brotherhood, yet in reality, as a scriptural author says, *sarva dharma samānam shāstra prayojanam*—"The aim of the scriptures of all religions is to perceive equality." By failing to realize this, we abuse the scriptures.

When God created the world, he had only one outlook and only one thought. In His creation, who is superior and who is inferior? Everyone has the same status in the court of God; He does not have different laws for people of different races and different persuasions. Everyone should learn to expand the feeling of universal brotherhood and mutual love; everyone should understand that one's fellow human beings are one's friends. As it is, people are slaying peace with their actions. Have they ever thought about whether the human race is progressing or falling? Can poisonous and destructive weapons help to spread peace? Is it not delusion to think that through them we will attain peace?

Once a group of tourists stopped in Nasrudin's town. Since Nasrudin happened to be standing in the public square, they asked him, "Are the people in this town friendly?"

"Of course," Nasrudin answered. "They're all good people. You can stay here without worrying."

One of the tourists noticed that Nasrudin had a gun slung around his neck and asked, "If the people here are so good, why do you have a gun around your neck?"

Nasrudin replied, "For my protection!"

This is exactly what we do in the name of peace. As long as the feeling that others are one's own does not become widespread, there will never be peace.

A Picture of the World

It is important for seekers to have a clear view of the world. Unless one perceives the world clearly, one has difficulty in perceiving its Lord. After one attains knowledge, one sees how the world appears to an enlightened being, but that attainment can come only after one has taken a look at the world.

The more civilized and educated a person considers himself to be, the more agitated he becomes. Other people may regard him as great and praise him, saying, "How much knowledge he has! What a writer! What a scholar!" Still, anxiety and difficulties follow him, and he is without peace. Why does his anxiety keep increasing? It increases because intellectual expansion is based on the notion of duality and difference, and as long as there is duality there can be no peace. Whereas the heart serves to unite, intellectual cleverness shatters one's awareness of equality. Only when such cleverness is eradicated can the inner mystery be experienced. The more deeply a person penetrates his heart, the less anxious he becomes. Science can grant power but not love, peace, kindness, or humanity. To attain these things one needs knowledge of the Self.

Now Jnaneshwar presents a picture of the world. One who assimilates this will become a real human being, a pure soul who knows true peace. These words occur in Lord Krishna's description of the characteristics of knowledge:

indriyārtheshu vairāgyamanahamkāra eva cha,
janma mrityu jarā vyādhi duhkha doshānudarshanam. [191]

"Indifference to the objects of the senses and also the absence of egoism and reflection on the evil of birth, death, old age, sickness, and pain."

"The mind of an enlightened being is completely detached from sense objects. Just as a person does not salivate at the sight of vomit, just as no one runs to embrace a dead man, swallows poison, enters a burning house, makes a tiger's cave his home, leaps into molten iron, or uses a python as a pillow, so an enlightened being is not

---

191. *Bhagavad Gita*, XIII, 8.

drawn to sense objects. He does not allow his senses to turn toward any objects, and his mind is indifferent to them. Although his body may be emaciated, he still maintains a strong desire to practice self-control. O Arjuna, all acts of penance have accumulated in him. He finds it as painful to live among people as to experience the final dissolution. He has a burning desire to practice yoga and dislikes the mere mention of others' company. He considers indulging in sense pleasures an evil to be rejected, like sleeping on a bed of arrows or wallowing in a mire of pus. He regards the pleasures of heaven as the rotten flesh of dogs. For him dispassion is the glory that enables him to attain the Self. An individual who has this kind of dispassion becomes worthy of enjoying the bliss of Brahman. Therefore, if you see that a person is completely detached from the pleasures of this world and the next, know that knowledge resides in him in its fullness.

"Just as a man with desires digs wells and builds bathing facilities for others to use, an enlightened being performs actions for the benefit of others but does not allow the pride of doership to touch his being. He performs religious rites and carries out the obligations that correspond to his station in life, but in him there is not the slightest feeling that he has performed any action. The wind blows in all places according to its nature. The sun shines with no sense of its own importance. The Vedas spontaneously give knowledge. The Ganges flows without a sense of purpose. Likewise, such a being performs his daily actions without pride. Just as trees bear fruit in due season but without the pride of giving fruit to others, all pride has been eradicated from the mind, deeds, and speech of an enlightened being. Although clouds float in the sky, the sky is untouched by them. In the same way, the body of an enlightened being performs actions, but he is detached from them just as the beads of a necklace are detached from each other when the string is removed.

"A drunkard is unaware of the clothes he is wearing, a clay statue is not conscious that it is holding a weapon, and a bull carrying scriptures on its back is ignorant of their content. Similarly, the ego of an enlightened being becomes completely useless; he is not even aware of it. The state of such a being is called selflessness. Without doubt, knowledge dwells in a person who lacks ego. He does not allow the pain of birth and death, disease and old age, or any other evils to touch his body. Remaining detached from them, he watches them just as a man with special powers protects himself from evil spirits, as yogis take precautions against obstacles, and as a mason makes use of a plumb line. In the same way, he watches death and disease without suffering their effects. He remembers his past sins just as a snake retains its feeling of enmity even from former births. The pain of past births continually gnaws at him, just as a grain of sand irritates the eye or an arrow gouges a wound. He always says, 'I fell into a pool of pus; I came out through the lowliest passage of the body. Alas! I relished the taste of sweat on the breast.' In this way, he is disgusted when he remembers his birth and resolves never to do anything that will make him take birth again. A gambler plays another game to make up for his losses. A son always looks for an opportunity to take revenge on an enemy of his father. One person runs after another to beat him and even the score between them. But an enlightened being wants only to wash his hands, and the same impulse makes him seek to break the bondage of birth. The shame of birth disturbs him, as dishonor continually distresses an eminent person.

"O Arjuna, if a swimmer is told that a river is deep in the middle, he either adjusts his garment while still on the bank or gives up the idea of swimming. A wise warrior prepares himself psychologically before he goes onto the battlefield and uses his shield to ward off blows before they strike him. If a traveler finds out that his next day's lodging will be in danger, he instantly takes precautions. Medicine is sent before a person dies. Similarly, a dispassionate being exercises immediate vigilance because he knows that whether it is today or at the end of an age, death must come one day. If a person is not on guard ahead of time, he is like someone staying in a burning house who has no time to dig a well for water. He fearfully remains where he is, just as a rock thrown into deep water lies there silently and no one listens to its cries. A man who is the enemy of another powerful man always keeps himself armed with weapons. A marriageable girl makes ready to leave her mother's house. A person who is going to take *sannyasa* prepares to give up the world. Likewise, an enlightened being remembers death before it comes and behaves accordingly. In this very lifetime, he puts an end to all future births, and then he lives only in his true nature. Such a person does not lack wisdom. Birth and death no longer harass him, and old age never touches his body; he retains his youthful enthusiasm.

"Such a being tells himself, 'Today my body looks very healthy and sturdy, but soon it will look like a withered vegetable. One day my hands and legs will become as tired and useless as a bankrupt business, and their strength will be like that of a king who has no prime minister to advise him. My nose, which now delights in the fragrance of flowers, will soon become as insensitive as a camel's knee. My head will be in the same condition as animals that contract a skin disease during the rainy season. Today my eyes compete with lotus petals, but they will soon become as dull as a dry gourd. My eyelids will hang like the dry bark of a tree, and my chest will waste away under the constant falling of tears. Just as a chameleon is sticky with the resin of a *babul* tree, my face will be smeared with saliva. Just as a kitchen sink is full of dirty water, my nose will be clogged with mucus. My lips are now rosy and I show my teeth when I laugh or speak eloquently, but from that same mouth saliva will flow. All my teeth will fall out, and my jaw will sag. Just as a farmer caught under the weight of debts or animals stuck in the mud after a rainstorm do not know how to extricate themselves, in the same way no matter how many millions of times I may try, I will not be able to move my tongue. Just as dry straws are blown away by the wind and fall at random on the ground, the hair on my head will also fall off. Just as rainwater pours down from the top of a mountain, rivers of saliva will flow from the window of my mouth. My speech will fail. My ears will lose their power of hearing. My entire body will look like a monkey's; it will tremble just as a straw scarecrow shakes when the wind blows. My legs will wobble when I walk, and my arms will become crooked and useless. My body will appear to be a travesty of its former state. I will no longer have control over the power of excretion, and people will wish that I would die and leave them alone. Seeing me, the entire world will spit on me, and I will have to plead with death again and again to come quickly and take me away. My relatives will become disgusted with me, women will call me a ghost, children will faint at the sight of me, and in this way I will become an object of loathing. When a coughing fit overcomes me, it will disturb my neighbors' sleep and they will say, "How many more people will that old man trouble?" '

"Therefore, while he is still young, a wise being thinks about the signs of old age, and the thought of it fills him with revulsion. Such a wise being tells himself, 'At the end, my body will be in this predicament. When my body is worn out from indulging in sense pleasures, what will remain of me to do *sadhana* in order to uplift myself?' He knows that before a person becomes deaf, he should listen to worthy teachings, and before his body becomes lame, he should go on pilgrimages. While his eyes have sight, he should see all that there is to see, and before his speech fails, he should speak sweetly. He knows very well that in the future his hands will be deformed, and that before this happens, he should use them for charity and good actions. He knows that when this wretched condition comes upon him, his mental state will deteriorate and that before he falls into this state, he should acquire pure knowledge. If a person discovers that thieves are going to come the next day and steal all his wealth, it is best for him to conceal his wealth immediately. A flame should be protected from the wind before it is blown out. When old age comes, this entire body will become useless, and for that reason one should become detached from it at once. If a traveler finds that there is no shelter ahead and sees dark clouds forming in the sky, he will be in danger if he disregards these things and leaves his house anyway. Similarly, it is useless to have a body in old age; there is no point in living for one hundred years. Pods of sesame seeds that have been threshed do not yield more seeds if threshed again. Fire cannot burn once it has become ashes. Even if a person lives one hundred years, he cannot do anything when he is old. A wise person bears in mind the thought of old age and tries when he is still young not to fall into its clutches. As long as he remains free of disease, he makes good use of his healthy body. Just as a wise person throws away a morsel of food that has fallen from a snake's mouth, he abandons attachment, which nourishes separation, pain, disaster, and distress. Filled with the bliss of the Self, he remains detached. With the help of self-restraint, he blocks all the doors of the senses through which sin enters the body. One who in this way works with great vigilance and control is the master of the wealth of knowledge."[192]

---

192. *Jnaneshwari*, XIII, 511–590.

The Essence of All Religions

Now I shall explain to you one more truth: the essence of all religions. Thus, you will be able to escape from the blindness of religion, perceive the Truth as it is, merge into it completely, and become happy.

At the end of the *Bhagavad Gita*, Shri Jagadguru Lord Krishna explains the essence of all religions and scriptures. This teaching is very mysterious and can be understood only by one with a sharp intellect. It is the Supreme Truth. Shri Krishna was omniscient, all-pervasive, and the benefactor and Self of all. In the *Shankara Bhashya* it is said:

sacchidānandarūpāya krishnāya klishtakārine,
namo vedānta vedyāya gurave buddhisākshine.

"His nature is *satchidananda*. He performs all actions spontaneously. He is perceived in the Upanishads at the end of the Vedas. He is the witness of the intellect of all and the Supreme Guru of all Gurus." My salutations to Shri Krishna Chandra, who is the Supreme Guru and who knows completely the *dharma* of the world. He is all-pervasive Consciousness. What final message does He give as the essence of the *Gita*? What does he say after explaining the essence of all religions? His statement is worthy of contemplation, for it is more mysterious than the mysterious. It is true and is the supreme mystery of life for those who seek knowledge of the Truth, who love God and desire to attain Him, and who have some understanding of life. The Lord says:

sarvadharmān parityajya māmekam sharanam vraja,
aham tvā sarvapāpebhyo mokshayishyāmi mā shuchaha.[193]

"Abandon all duties and take refuge in Me alone. I will liberate you from all sins. Do not grieve."

"Just as desire gives rise to sorrow, criticizing others causes sin, and misfortune brings about poverty, so igno-

---

193. *Bhagavad Gita*, XVIII, 66.

rance is the source of good or evil actions, which in turn lead one to heaven or hell. Through the knowledge of the Self, rid yourself of all the fantasies created by ignorance. The delusion of mistaking a rope for a snake vanishes when you pick up the rope. When a dream ends, all the activities of the dream also cease. The moon loses its yellow hue once one's jaundice is cured, and the bitter taste in one's mouth automatically disappears when one recovers from a disease. A mirage disappears when the sun sinks over the horizon, and there is no possibility of fire after the wood is removed. In the same way, cast out ignorance, which is the root of good and evil actions and which creates havoc. Once you eradicate ignorance, the conflict between religion and irreligion ceases. Once ignorance is dispelled, I alone remain, just as when sleeping and dreaming are over, only you exist. When nothing is left except Me, the individual soul merges into My own Self. To take refuge in Me is to eliminate any difference between you and Me and to become one with Me. When a pot is destroyed, the space within the pot merges into the space outside, and in the same way through surrender you become one with Me. Just as a gold ball merges into gold and waves merge into water, O Arjuna, take refuge in Me and merge into Me. Give up fantasies which resemble the idea that the fire beneath the sea has swallowed the ocean and then burned it. It is absurd to say that your individuality is not obliterated after you have taken refuge in Me; an intellect that produces such notions should be ashamed. O Arjuna, even if a simple serving maid becomes a king's consort, she obtains the grandeur of a kingdom. So do not listen to such nonsense as the idea that even after union with Me, the knot of individuality is not loosened. You can serve Me very easily by becoming one with Me; serve Me in that way, for it is the only means of attaining knowledge. Once butter has been churned from milk, you cannot blend the butter back into the milk even if you try a million times. In the same way, once you take refuge in Me with the awareness of unity, the conflict between religion and irreligion cannot touch you. If iron lies out in the open it rusts, but if it comes in contact with the philosophers' stone it becomes gold and cannot rust. Once fire has been kindled from two pieces of wood, the fire cannot remain concealed in the wood. O Arjuna, can the sun ever see darkness? Can one have the delusion of seeing a dream in the waking state? In the same way, after a person becomes one with Me, what is left except My own nature? Therefore, never think of anyone but Me. I become all your virtues and sins. All bondage and sin are the result of the sense of duality and are destroyed once knowledge of Me is attained. O wise Arjuna, a grain of salt that falls into water becomes the water, and in the same way if you take refuge in Me completely, with one-pointed devotion, you will become Me. O Arjuna, when you become one with Me, you will automatically become liberated. Accept Me. With My light, I will free you. Therefore, O Arjuna, have no more anxiety. O wise Arjuna, knowing Me, take refuge in Me alone."

Shri Krishna, the witness of all, the all-pervasive One, whose form was the universe, said these things to Arjuna. Then, stretching out His right arm, dark-skinned and adorned with bracelets, He embraced Arjuna, the best among all devotees. In order to grant Arjuna the experience of that state from which speech, unable to reach it, returns carrying the intellect, that state which is unattainable through word or thought, Shri Krishna drew Arjuna toward Him under the pretext of a mere embrace. When Arjuna's heart touched that of Shri Krishna, the secret of Shri Krishna's heart entered Arjuna's heart. When Arjuna's notion of duality departed, Shri Krishna made Arjuna merge into Him. Although there had been duality, Shri Krishna made Arjuna one with Him, like one lamp kindled by another. At that moment, great joy flooded Arjuna's heart, and the Lord, in spite of His strength, was submerged in it. If one ocean merges into another, the mass of water is doubled and begins to leap into the sky. In the same way, during the union of Shri Krishna and Arjuna, their joy knew no bounds. Who can describe that union? The whole universe was filled with the Lord. [194]

An Exposition of the Bhagavad Gita

In this way, Shri Krishna revealed the *Bhagavad Gita*, the essence of the Vedas and the holiest of all the authoritative treatises. You may wonder how the *Gita* was the origin of the Vedas. I will explain that to you also. Mahavishnu, from whose breath all the Vedas sprang, speaks the truth of the *Gita* from His own mouth. For that reason, the *Gita* can be said to be the source of the Vedas. It can also be explained in another way: That which is imperishable and conceals its own expansion within itself should be considered the seed of the Vedas. Just as a seed contains a tree, in the same way the *Gita* contains the three sections [195] of the Vedas. Therefore, it seems clear to me that the *Gita* is the seed of the Vedas. The three sections of the Vedas adorn the *Gita* just as the body is adorned with diamonds, rubies, and other jewels.

Now I will explain to you the places in which each of the three branches of the Vedas are located. The first chapter of the *Gita* is an introduction to the general teaching of the *Gita*, while the second chapter reveals the meaning of the Sankhya philosophy, explaining that to attain liberation one needs only knowledge of that and nothing else. The third chapter describes the means of attaining liberation for those who are bound by ignorance. It tells how a person should abandon all sense of individuality and all

---

194. *Jnaneshwari*, XVIII, 1381-1415.
195. Known as *karma kanda* (works), *deva kanda* (worship), and *jnana kanda* (knowledge).

action arising from desire and should faultlessly carry out all his prescribed duties. The third chapter, in which the Lord teaches that one should perform actions with pure feeling, is called *karma kanda*, the chapter concerning work. Now how can the performance of one's daily duty and periodic actions break the bondage of ignorance and make one a seeker? The Lord explains that one should perform all one's actions while offering them to Brahman, the Absolute, that all prescribed actions carried out through the body, speech, or mind should be directed toward God. At the end of the fourth chapter, the delicious dish of karma yoga performed through devotion to God is served. Then, until the end of the eleventh chapter, in which there is the vision of the cosmic form, the service to God through action is described. In these eight chapters, the worship of deities, which is called *deva kanda*, is explained. I am eliminating all your confusion by telling you what the *Gita* says. Through devotion to God and His grace, one attains from the Guru the divine knowledge, filled with love, which has come down through the Guru's lineage. The twelfth chapter describes how a person can increase his knowledge and love and become free of hatred and pride, while the twelfth through the fifteenth chapters expound the ripening of the fruit of knowledge. These four chapters, the last of which describes the tree with its roots growing upward, deal with knowledge, *jnana kanda*.

Thus, in the exposition given in these three sections of the *Gita*, the Vedas are found in a beautiful form adorned with the jewels of the verses of the *Gita*. The three sections of the Vedas proclaim the fruit of liberation and insist that it must be attained. All the forms of ignorance, which are in constant conflict with the knowledge leading to liberation, are discussed in the sixteenth chapter. The theme of the seventeenth chapter is that with the scriptures as one's companion, all enemies can be overcome. In this way, from the first chapter to the end of the seventeenth, the

Lord has explained the mystery of the Vedas. Finally, the essence of all seventeen chapters is given in the eighteenth, which is the culmination of all the preceding chapters.

In the extraordinary generosity with which it gives the knowledge of one's own Self, the *Bhagavad Gita* contains the essence of the Vedas. The Vedas are filled with the wealth of knowledge, yet they are more miserly than anyone. For only *brahmins*, warriors, and businessmen can listen to them; women and members of the lower castes are not given a place in the temple of Vedic knowledge. Therefore, I feel that in order to remove this ancient defect, the Vedas have taken the form of the *Bhagavad Gita* and thus become available to everyone. In the form of the *Gita*, the meaning of the Vedas enters the mind. Through the sense of hearing it reaches the ears, and through repetition it dwells on the tongue. In this way, it has become accessible to all. The Vedas in the form of the *Gita* give the bliss of liberation to those who memorize it, while even to those ordinary people who copy the *Gita* and keep it with them in book form, the Vedas have opened the bliss of liberation like a stall that gives travelers free food at the crossroads. The sky is free to all who live in the air, and the earth to all who dwell on it. The light of the sun in the heavens can be enjoyed by all without restrictions. Similarly, the *Bhagavad Gita* is the same for everyone without limitations. No matter who turns to it, it accepts him, considering him neither high nor low. Without any sense of duality, the *Bhagavad Gita* gives the joy of liberation to all and bestows peace on the entire world. The Vedas, ashamed of their old defect, were reborn in the womb of the *Gita*, whose fame has now become pure and bright. In this way, the *Gita*, which was expounded by Krishna to Arjuna, is a form of the Vedas that is available to all. A cow's udder is filled with love for the sake of its calf, yet it supplies milk to the entire household. In the same way, for the sake of Arjuna, the *Gita* has uplifted the entire world. Taking compassion on the thirsty *chataka* bird, the clouds send down rain, but the entire animate and inanimate creation benefits from that water. The sun rises every day for the sake of the lotuses that depend on it, but the entire world derives joy from it. Similarly, by revealing the *Bhagavad Gita* for Arjuna, the Lord removed the burden of the entire world. The Lord is not just the husband of Lakshmi. The *Gita* is like the sun in the heavens which, in the form of Krishna's mouth, illuminates for the world the jewels of all the scriptures. Blessed is the family of Arjuna, for he has been found worthy of receiving this knowledge and has opened the door of the *Gita* to the entire world.

After His union with Arjuna, Sadguru Shri Krishna restored his sense of separateness and asked, "O Arjuna, were you pleased with this scripture?" Arjuna said, "Yes, Lord, through the blessings of Your grace, I found it perfect." Then the Lord again began to speak: "O Arjuna, to obtain the hidden treasure, one needs exceptional strength of destiny. Only a rare being obtains the great fortune of enjoying that treasure. What efforts the gods and demons had to put forth to churn the ocean of pure milk! All their efforts eventually bore fruit, because the churners saw with their own eyes the nectar that came from it. But because they did not distribute it correctly, that which was given to them to bring immortality brought about their death. If a person accumulates wealth without knowing how to enjoy it, it leads to misfortune. King Nahusha became the lord of heaven, but since he did not know how to conduct himself there, he was changed into a serpent. O Arjuna, because you have acquired countless merits, you have become worthy of receiving the teachings of the best of all scriptures. Now follow these teachings completely and with unswerving faith. Otherwise, O Arjuna, if you do not pay sufficient attention to this divine knowledge which has come down through the lineage of the Guru, and if you only perform religious rites, you will be in the same condition as those gods who churned the ocean. You may possess a fine, healthy, and beautiful cow, but you can drink its milk in the evening only if you know the art of milking it. Similarly, know that when the Guru becomes pleased the disciple attains knowledge, but that knowledge bears fruit only when the disciple properly follows the path shown by the Guru. Therefore, follow with great faith the divine teaching which has come down from the lineage of the Guru."[196]

Our time is different from the orthodox era when certain people were prohibited from studying the scriptures. Even in Vedic times, the yogini Gargi went to the place where King Janaka performed fire sacrifices and entered into a great discussion with the sage Yajnavalkya. More recently, the sage Dayananda broke the bonds of the orthodox attitude toward women and people of the lower castes. Then Mahatma Gandhiji made all castes equal and gave the untouchables the name of *harijan*, the people of God. It is obvious that the orthodox restrictions are not applied in Siddha Yoga Dham; everyone chants the *Rudram*, which is a portion of the *Rig Veda*. Everyone should read and understand the scriptures. By performing good actions, a person should make himself a pure temple of God and worship the Lord of the Self within.

The Praise of the Guru

This book began with the Guru-disciple relationship, and now it will end with the Guru's praises.

Salutations to that resplendent sun, the Sadguru, which has risen, dispelling the illusion of the universe and causing the lotus of nonduality to open its petals. He swallows up the night of ignorance, removes the moon-

---

196. *Jnaneshwari*, XVIII, 1416-1474.

light of the duality of knowledge and ignorance, and ushers in the day of Self-knowledge for the wise. When that sun rises, the birds of individual souls attain the vision of the knowledge of the Self and leave the nests of their bodies. When the sun rises, the bee of Consciousness, enclosed in the lotus of desires which is the body, is suddenly set free. On the opposite bank of the river of duality, which springs from the conflicting teachings of the scriptures, intellect and understanding, crying out like a pair of geese in the distress of their separation, are granted the awareness of equality. The sun of the Guru lights up the sky of the space of Consciousness, just as a lamp illumines a house. At the rising of the sun, the thieves' night of duality passes away, and travelers along the path of yoga begin to experience the Self. Touched by its rays of discrimination, the sparks of the sun crystal of the intellect burst into flame and burn down the forests of worldly existence. The network of its scorching rays settles over the land of the Self, and the mirage of the flood of psychic powers rises. When the sun reaches the height of the wisdom of the Self, it begins to blaze in the afternoon of union with the Absolute, and then the shadow of the individual self disappears. When the night of illusion is over, there is no room for the appearance of the world or for the sleep of wrong knowledge. In this way, in the city of the knowledge of unity, only joy and nothing but joy exists, and the give-and-take of worldly pleasures ceases. The light of the sun gives the perpetual daylight of liberation. The sun of the Guru is the monarch of the sky of the Self, and when he rises the process of rising and setting and all the ten directions disappear. He destroys the duality of knowledge and ignorance and clearly reveals to his disciples their hidden principle, the Self. What more can be said? In this way, the sun brings about a new and extraordinary dawn.

Who can see the sun of knowledge, which is beyond both day and night? To him who is a self-luminous sphere of light, the enlightened Nivrittinath, I bow down again and again. If I begin to praise him with words, I will discover the weakness of my speech. Only when the glory of a deity is imprinted on the heart and has become one with the intellect can he be praised properly. That can be understood only when the notion of the names and forms of all objects is completely destroyed and can be truly described only by embracing silence. It is experienced by an individual who becomes one with it. While one is describing the characteristics of the Guru, all four levels of speech—*pashyanti* and *madhyama*, together with *para* and *vaikhari*—disappear. O Guru! As your servant, I mentally adorn you with the hymns of words. To say that you accept this adornment will create an obstacle to the bliss of unity. A beggar becomes astounded when he sees the ocean of nectar, forgets his worthiness or lack of worthiness, and honors the ocean by offering vegetables to it. In such a case, the ocean of nectar should appreciate the offering of vegetables, taking account only of the joy and enthusiasm of the beggar. Similarly, if you hide your divine effulgence and acknowledge my ordinary lamp of devotion, then I will be completely fulfilled. If a child knew right from wrong, how could he experience childhood? His mother delights in his childishness. If the water from the streets flows into the Ganges, will the Ganges say, "No, don't come with me. Go away"? Brigu committed such a serious offense when he kicked the Lord, yet Krishna, the wielder of the Sharnga bow, accepted it gladly and considered the footprint to be an ornament. If the sky filled with dark clouds appears before the sun, does the sun offend the sky by saying, "Get out of here"? O Guru, please bear with me if I have become involved in the knowledge of duality and have weighed you on the scale of comparison with the sun. As you have borne with those who saw you in their meditation and *samadhi*, and with the Vedas which have described you, in the same way please be patient with me and equally just.

O Lord, today I have delighted in extolling your merits. Please do not blame me. Do what you like, but as long as I am not completely satisfied and my life is not finished, I will not stop praising you. I have acquired twice my usual strength as a result of my supreme fortune in describing with great enthusiasm the nectar of the *Bhagavad Gita* of Shri Guru. My tongue must have practiced the austerity of correct speech for many lifetimes, O Guru, and now is obtaining the infinite fruit of that penance. I must have performed extraordinary deeds of merit, the results of which have today given me the intellect to praise you and to finish my work. I had entered the forest of individuality and become trapped in the village of death. Today that predicament has come to an end because I have been allowed to describe your fame, which is known by the name of the *Bhagavad Gita* and which has destroyed the notion of the world. If Mahalakshmi, great prosperity, comes to dwell in the house of a poor man, how can he be called poor? If through good fortune the sun comes as a guest to the house of darkness, will not that darkness become the light of the world? The universe is not even a speck compared to the greatness of God. If that Lord is carried away by the waves of His devotees' love, what form will He not take for the sake of those devotees? For me to expound the *Bhagavad Gita*, which is like the Guru, is as impossible as trying to smell the fragrance of a flower in the sky. But you have power, and through that you have fulfilled my desire.[197]

Shri Guru is the source of all *sadhanas*, all religions, and all happiness. One can attain the grandeur of the entire world by receiving a single drop of his compassion. This book concerns the relationship between the Guru and the disciple. When I first read about Jnaneshwar's devotion to the Guru, in the section of *Jnaneshwari* on service to the Guru

---

197. Ibid., XVI, 1, 39.

as well as in the various other sections concerning the Guru, my faith in the Guru became very firm, and I attained supreme devotion and inner love for him. Because of that love, the Guru is present everywhere for me. You may wonder why a person who has faith in the Self takes so much interest in the Guru. I can only say that if you are fortunate enough, you will understand this and will know who the Guru is. The Guru is the Self, God, the One who pervades all animate beings and inanimate objects, the Supreme Principle, and absolute bliss.

O Gurudev, you are my Self, supreme bliss. Through your inspiration, I have written this. You alone will read it, you who live within everyone and are experienced as the Self. O compassionate and merciful one! Even *samadhi* is petty compared to the extraordinary experience of your inner love. From you alone one attains interest in attaining the bliss of the Self. You are all, and all are you. *Om guru, jaya guru.* O Shri Guru, I hail you. *Sadgurunāth mahārāj ki jay!*

GLOSSARY

Abhisheka: A ritual bath given to a deity or idol.

Arati: The waving of lights, incense, camphor, and other auspicious materials as an act of worship.

Arjuna: A famous warrior and one of the heroes of the *Mahabharata* epic. It was to Arjuna that Krishna imparted the knowledge of the *Bhagavad Gita*.

Asana: (1) Any one of various bodily postures practiced to strengthen the body, purify the nerves, and develop one-pointedness of mind; the yoga texts describe eighty-four major *asanas*. (2) A seat or mat on which one sits for meditation.

Ashram: An institution or community where spiritual discipline is practiced; the abode of a saint or holy man.

Baba: A term of affection for a saint or holy man.

Bandha (lit. lock): A type of hatha yoga position practiced to keep the *prana* from flowing out of the body.

Bartruhari: A king who renounced his kingdom to become a yogi; writer of many moral and spiritual poems.

Bhagavad Gita: A portion of the *Mahabharata* and one of the great works of spiritual literature, in which Lord Krishna explains the path of liberation to Arjuna on the battlefield of the war described in the epic poem.

Bhagawan: Lord; one who is glorious, illustrious, divine, venerable.

Bhairava: A name of Shiva meaning the Lord who is responsible for the creation, sustenance, and dissolution of the universe.

Bhakti Sutras: Definitive treatise on love and devotion to God; composed by the sage Narada.

Brahma: The creator of the universe.

Brahman: Vedantic term for the Absolute Reality.

Brahmin: The first caste of Hindu society, the members of which were by tradition priests, scholars, and teachers.

Caste: Ancient Indian society was organized into four *varnas* (divisions, or castes): *brahmins* (scholars, priests, and teachers); *kshatriyas* (rulers and warriors); *vaishyas* (business and agricultural classes); and *shudras* (menial laborers).

Chakora bird: A bird that feeds on the dew of the moon.

Chakra (lit. wheel): In the human body, there are seven major energy centers, or nerve plexes, called *chakras*, which are located in the subtle body.

Chandika: One of the forms of the Divine Mother.

Chataka bird: A bird that feeds on rainwater.

Chit Shakti: (1) The power of self-revelation by which the Supreme shines by itself. (2) Universal Consciousness.

Darshan: (1) Spiritual philosophy. (2) Seeing God, an image of God, or a holy being.

Dharma: Righteousness; religion; the path to Truth.

Dhoti: Common dress for men in India; a length of material wrapped around the waist.

Ekanath Maharaj (1528-1609): Householder poet-saint· of Maharashtra. The illustrious disciple of Janardan Swami, he was renowned in his later life for his scriptural commentaries and spiritual poetry.

Five causes of action: (1) The body; (2) the reflection of Consciousness which identifies itself as the doer—that is, the individual self; (3) the senses, including the mind; (4) the vital airs; and (5) the intellect and the deities (presiding forces) of the senses.

Five elements: Ether, air, fire, water, earth. From these, the whole material creation is composed.

Five organs of action: The powers of speaking, grasping, locomotion, procreation, and excretion.

Five senses of perception: Hearing, seeing, touching, tasting, and smelling.

Four types of liberation: (1) *Sayujya*, total absorption in Brahman; (2) *salokya*, living as a subject in the kingdom of God; (3) *samipya*, being very close to God physically; and (4) *sarupya*, assuming a form similar to God's.

Garuda: The mount of Lord Vishnu.

Ghee: Clarified butter.

Gorakhnath: One of the nine Naths, a lineage of yogis known for their extraordinary powers. Gorakhnath was the Guru of Gahininath, who initiated Nivrittinath, Jnaneshwar's older brother and Guru.

Gunas: The three basic qualities of nature, which determine the inherent characteristics of all created things. They are *sattva*—purity, light, harmony; *rajas*—activity, passion; and *tamas*—dullness, inertia, ignorance.

Guru: A spiritual master who has attained oneness with God, who initiates his disciples and devotees into the spiritual path and guides them to liberation.

Gurudev: A term of address for the Guru, signifying that he is considered a deity.

Guru Gita (lit. song of the Guru): A garland of mantras in the form of a dialogue between Shiva and His consort Parvati, which explains the identity of the Guru with the Supreme Absolute and describes the nature of the Guru, the Guru-disciple relationship, and meditation on the Guru.

Hatha yoga: A yogic discipline by which the *samadhi* state is attained through union of the *prana* and *apana* (ingoing and outgoing breath). Various bodily and mental exercises are practiced in order to purify the *nadis* and bring about the even flow of *prana*. When the flow of *prana* is even, the mind becomes still. One then experiences equality-consciousness and enters into the state of *samadhi*.

Ida and *pingala*: *Nadis* located in the spinal column in the subtle body, on either side of the *sushumna*. The *ida* is known as the moon *nadi* and is on the left side. The *pingala* is known as the sun *nadi* and is on the right side. *See also Nadi.*

Jain: An Indian sect that follows strict nonviolence.

Jalandhara bandha: A yogic lock in which the chin is pressed to the chest. *See also Bandha.*

Jnaneshwar Maharaj (1275-1296): Foremost among the saints of Maharashtra and a child yogi of extraordinary powers. He was born into a family of saints, and his older brother Nivrittinath was his Guru. His verse commentary on the *Bhagavad Gita*, the *Jnaneshwari*, written in the Marathi language, is acknowledged as one of the most important spiritual works. He took live *samadhi* at the age of 21 in Alandi, where his *samadhi* shrine continues to attract thousands of seekers.

Kabir (1440-1518): A great poet-saint who lived his life as a weaver in Benares. His followers were both Hindus and Moslems, and his influence was a strong force in overcoming religious factionalism.

Kailasa: A mountain peak in the Himalayas (in present-day Tibet) revered as the abode of Shiva.

Kamakshi Tantra: An important tantric work. *See also* Tantra.

Karma: Physical, mental, or verbal action.

Kashmir Shaivism: Nondual philosophy that recognizes the entire universe as a manifestation of Chiti, or divine conscious energy. Kashmir Shaivism explains how the formless, unmanifest Supreme Principle manifests as the universe. The authoritative scripture of Kashmir Shaivism is the *Shiva Sutras*.

Krishna (lit. the dark one; the one who attracts irresistibly): The eighth incarnation of Vishnu, whose life story is described in the *Shrimad Bhagavatam* and the *Mahabharata* and whose spiritual teachings are contained in the *Bhagavad Gita*.

Kularnava Tantra: A great tantric treatise; the basic work of Kaula Tantricism. *See also* Tantra.

Kum-kum: A red powder used in Hindu worship and worn as an auspicious mark on the foreheads of married women and *sadhus*.

Kundalini (lit. coiled one): The primordial Shakti, or cosmic energy, that lies coiled in the *muladhara chakra* of every individual. When awakened, Kundalini begins to move upward within the *sushumna*, the subtle central channel, piercing the *chakras* and initiating various yogic processes which bring about total purification and rejuvenation of the entire being. When Kundalini enters the *sahasrara*, the spiritual center in the crown of the head, the individual self merges in the universal Self and attains the state of Self-realization.

Lakshmi: Goddess of wealth and fortune; wife of Lord Vishnu.

Levels of speech: Sound originates in the deepest level of unmanifest Consciousness, the *para* level. From here, it rises successively through the *pashyanti* level to the *madhyama* (subtle) level of speech until it manifests on the gross level as *vaikhari*, or articulated speech. The four levels of speech correspond to the four bodies—*vaikhari* to the gross body, *madhyama* to the subtle body, *pashyanti* to the causal body, and *para* to the supracausal body.

Liberation: Freedom from the cycle of birth and death; state of realization of oneness with the Absolute.

Mahabharata: An epic poem composed by the sage Vyasa which recounts the struggle between the Kaurava and the Pandava brothers over a disputed kingdom. As its vast narrative unfolds, a storehouse of Indian secular and religious lore is revealed. The *Bhagavad Gita* occurs in the latter portion of the *Mahabharata*.

Mahavishnu: The Supreme Reality (*see* Vishnu).

Mahishasura (lit. great demon): A demon in the form of a buffalo, who fought the Goddess Chandika and was defeated by her.

Mantra: Cosmic word or divine sound; a name of God.

Mantra virya: The perfect "I"-consciousness, which is the fountainhead of all the powers or potencies behind the mantra; Shiva-consciousness; the experience of *paravak* (sound as pure Consciousness).

Matruka: Letter or sound syllable which is the basis of all words and hence of all knowledge; Shakti in sound form that manifests the universe. Because it is the source of words, *matruka* is the source of ignorance (which comes about mainly through the ideas produced by words).

Maya: The force that shows the unreal as real and presents that which is temporary and short-lived as permanent and everlasting.

Mira (1433-1468): A queen and poet-saint famous for her poems of devotion to Krishna. She was so absorbed in her love for Krishna that when she was given poison by disapproving relatives, she drank it considering it Krishna and was not harmed.

Mount Meru: A sacred mountain in the Himalayas which is always covered with snow.

Mudra virya: The power by which one experiences the emergence of the supreme "I"-consciousness; also called *mantra virya* or the *khechari* state.

Muladhara: Spiritual center at the base of the spine where the Kundalini lies dormant.

Mullah: A Muslim priest.

Nada: Metaphysically, the first movement of Shiva-Shakti toward manifestation. In yoga, the unstruck sound experienced in meditation.

Nadi: Subtle channel within the body through which *prana* flows.

Nanak (also known as Guru Nanak, Nanakdev; 1469-1538): The founder and first Guru of the Sikh religion. He traveled widely, teaching liberal religious and social doctrines.

Narada: A divine *rishi*, or seer, who was a great devotee and servant of Vishnu. He appears in many of the Puranas and is the author of the *Narada Bhakti Sutras*, the authoritative text on bhakti yoga.

Narayana: A name for Vishnu; often depicted as reclining on the milky ocean with the serpent Shesha as his couch.

Nasrudin: A comic character who is the hero of many Sufi teaching stories.

Naths: A lineage of yogis known for their extraordinary powers.

Nivrittinath: The elder brother and Guru of Jnaneshwar Maharaj.

Om namah shivaya: A mantra meaning "salutations to Shiva"; Shiva denotes the inner Self. It is known as the great redeeming mantra because it has the power to grant worldly fulfillment as well as spiritual realization.

Parashiva: The Ultimate Reality; the core of all.

Paravani: The deepest level of sound; the level of the Supreme Consciousness from which all sound emanates.

Parvati (lit. daughter of the mountains): Wife of Shiva and daughter of the King of the Himalayas; a name of the Universal Mother or Shakti.

Patanjali: A great sage and author of the *Yoga Sutras*.

Philosophers' stone: A jewel that is said to have the power to transmute base metals into gold.

Prakruti: Primordial nature, the natural force that manifests the universe; also, the world of matter. In Kashmir Shaivism, *prakruti* is identified with Shakti.

Prana: Vital force; also the inhalation in the breathing process. Within the body, there are five major *pranas—prana, apana, viyana, udana,* and *samana.*

Pranayama: The regulation and restraint of breath.

Prasad: A divine gift; often used to refer to food that is offered to God and is thus considered blessed.

Pratyabhijnahridayam (lit. the heart of the doctrine of recognition): A concise treatise of twenty *sutras* by Kshemaraja which summarizes the Pratyabhijna philosophy of Kashmir Shaivism. In essence it states that we have forgotten our true nature by identifying with the body. Realization is a process of recognizing our true Self. Swami Muktananda has commented on some of these *sutras* in his books *Siddha Meditation* and *Secret of the Siddhas. See also* Kashmir Shaivism.

Puranas (lit. ancient legends): Sacred books containing stories, legends, and hymns about the creation of the universe, the incarnations of God, and the instructions of various deities, as well as the spiritual legacies of ancient sages and kings. There are eighteen Puranas.

Purusha: The individual soul; the form of the Supreme Principle that resides within a human being. In Kashmir Shaivism, the *purusha* is identified with Shiva.

Rajas: Activity or passion (one of the three *gunas*).

Rama: The eighth incarnation of Vishnu, whose life story is told in the *Ramayana* epic; a name of the all-pervasive Supreme Reality.

Sacred thread: Thread worn over one shoulder indicating the religious initiation of the *brahmin, kshatriya,* and *vaishya* castes.

Sadguru: A true Guru. *See* Guru.

Sadhana: The practice of spiritual discipline.

Sadhu: Holy man or spiritual seeker.

Sahasrara: Thousand-petaled spiritual center at the crown of the head where one experiences the highest states of consciousness.

Sahib: A term of respectful address.

Samadhi: A state of meditative union with the Absolute.

Sankhya: An important philosophical school founded by the sage Kapilamuni, which views the world as composed of two ultimate realities: spirit (*purusha*) and matter (*prakriti*). Self-realization consists of understanding the distinction between *purusha* (the observer) and *prakriti* (the observed).

Sannyasa: The fourth stage of traditional Indian life; the time of complete renunciation in which one is freed from all worldly obligations and responsibilities in order to devote one's life to the pursuit of Self-realization.

Satchidananda: The nature of the Supreme Reality. *Sat* is being, that which exists in all times, in all places, and in all things; *chit* is consciousness, that which illumines all places, times, and things; *ananda* is absolute bliss.

Satsang: A meeting of devotees for the purpose of listening to scriptural readings, chanting, or sitting in the presence of a holy being; the company of saints and devotees.

Sattva: Purity (one of the three *gunas*).

Seven components: Bone, flesh, marrow, fat, blood, lymphatic fluid, sexual fluid.

Shakti (also known as Chiti, Kundalini, Kundalini Shakti): The divine cosmic power which projects, maintains, and dissolves the universe.

Shaktipat: The transmission of spiritual power (Shakti) from the Guru to the disciple; spiritual awakening by grace.

Shankara: A name for Shiva.

Shankaracharya (788-820): One of the greatest of India's philosophers and sages, who expounded the philosophy of absolute nondualism (Advaita Vedanta). In addition to his writing and teaching, he established *maths* (ashrams) in the four corners of India.

Shesha: Divine serpent who, according to Puranic legend, holds the earth on his mantle.

Shiva: (1) A name for the all-pervasive Supreme Reality. (2) One of the Hindu trinity, representing God as the destroyer; the personal God of the Shaivites. In His personal form, He is portrayed as a yogi wearing a tiger skin and holding a trident, with snakes coiled around His neck and arms.

Shiva Sutras: A Sanskrit text which Shiva revealed to the sage Vasuguptacharya. It consists of seventy-seven *sutras*, which were found inscribed on a rock in Kashmir. It is the major scriptural authority for the philosophical school of Kashmir Shaivism.

Shree: A term of respect; also wealth, prosperity, glory, success; possessor of all these.

Siddha: A perfected yogi; one who has attained the highest state and become one with the Absolute.

Siddha Yoga: The yoga which takes place spontaneously within a seeker whose Kundalini has been awakened by a Siddha Guru and which leads to the state of spiritual perfection.

Six enemies: Desire, lust, greed, anger, envy, and pride.

So'ham (lit. I am That): The natural vibration of the Self, which occurs spontaneously with each incoming and outgoing breath. By becoming aware of it, a yogi experiences the identity between his individual self and the Supreme Self.

Sunderdas (1596-1689): A renowned Hindu poet-saint born in Rajasthan.

Sutra: An aphorism, or pithy saying.

Tamas: Inertia or dullness (one of the three gunas).

Tantra: An esoteric spiritual discipline in which Shakti, the creative power of the Absolute, is worshipped as the Divine Mother through the practice of rituals, mantras, and yantras (visual symbols). The goal of tantra is attaining Self-realization through Kundalini awakening and through uniting the two principles Shiva and Shakti.

Tattva (lit. that-ness): That which is the essence of each stage of manifestation. The process of creation, according to Kashmir Shaivism, contains thirty-six tattvas: Shiva, Shakti, Sadashiva, Ishwara, shuddha vidya, maya tattva, the five cloaks (pancha kanchukas), purusha (individual soul), prakriti (primordial nature, the basic stuff of the material universe), buddhi (intellect), ahamkara (ego), manas (mind), the five senses of perception, the five powers of action, the five tanmatras, or rudimentary elements, and the five gross elements. These comprise the creation from Shiva to the earth. For more information see Introduction to Kashmir Shaivism (Oakland, California: SYDA Foundation, 1978).

Three bodily humors: Wind, bile, and phlegm.

Three fires: Three fires that lie at the center of the earth and burst into flame at the time of cosmic dissolution, engulfing the entire world.

Tukaram Maharaj (1608-1650): Great poet-saint of Maharashtra; author of thousands of abhangas (devotional songs).

Tulasidas (1532-1623): North Indian poet-saint and author of Ramacharitamanas, the life story of Lord Rama written in Hindi, which is still one of the most popular scriptures in India.

Uddiyana bandha: A yogic lock in which the stomach muscles are drawn inward. See also Bandha.

Upanishads: The teachings of the ancient sages which form the knowledge or end portion of the Vedas. The central teaching of the Upanishads is that the Self of a human being is the same as Brahman, the Absolute. The goal of life, according to the Upanishads, is realization of Brahman.

Vaikuntha: The divine abode of Lord Vishnu.

Vajra bandha (also known as mula bandha): A yogic lock in which the sphincter muscles are drawn upward and contracted. See also Bandha.

Vajra posture: A meditation posture in which the knees are placed together, the legs are folded underneath, and one sits on one's heels. See also Bandha.

Vedanta: A philosophical school founded by Badarayana, which contains the philosophical teachings of the Upanishads and investigates the nature and relationship of the Absolute, the world, and the Self.

Vedas: Very ancient and authoritative revealed scriptures of India.

Vedavyasa (Vyasa): One of the greatest sages of Indian tradition, who is held to be the compiler of the Vedas and Puranas, as well as the author of the *Mahabharata*.

Vishnu: (1) A name for the all-pervasive Supreme Reality. (2) One of the Hindu trinity, representing God as the sustainer; the personal God of the Vaishnavas. In His personal form, He is portrayed as four-armed and holding a conch, a discus, a lotus, and a mace. He is dark blue. During times of great wickedness and trouble, Vishnu incarnates on the earth in order to protect human beings and gods and reestablish righteousness. There are ten such incarnations in our present world cycle, Rama and Krishna being the most important.

Vishnu Sahasranam: A hymn composed of one thousand names of Vishnu; found in the *Mahabharata*. Chanting this hymn is considered to be one of the most effective spiritual practices.

Vishuddha: The *chakra* located in the throat.

Vitthal (lit. the place of the brick): Krishna went to the house of Pundalik, who asked Him to wait while he tended to his aging parents and threw a brick for Him to stand on. The form of Krishna standing on a brick is known as Vitthal. His image is enshrined in Pandharpur, a famous place of pilgrimage in Maharashtra, and was worshipped by the poet-saints of Maharashtra and Karnataka.

Void: (1) The state of nothingness experienced in deep sleep. (2) The state of the formless Absolute. According to the Buddhists, this is a state of nonexistence. In Kashmir Shaivism, however, Void is emptiness in the sense that it is without manifest creation. It is not a state of nonexistence, because it has the nature of being, consciousness, and bliss.

Yajnavalkya: A sage whose teachings are recorded in the *Brihadaranyaka Upanishad*.

Yamas and *niyamas*: Restraints (*yamas*) and observances (*niyamas*) that are considered vital to one who is pursuing a yogic life. *Yamas* consist of abstention from violence, falsehood, theft, and acquisitiveness, as well as the vow of celibacy. *Niyamas* include purity, contentment, observance of austerities, self-study, and self-surrender.

Yoga (lit. union): The state of oneness with the Self, God; the practices leading to that state.

Yoga Sutras: Patanjali's treatise on yoga; one of the six philosophies of India and the authoritative text on raja yoga.

INDEX

OTHER PUBLICATIONS

BY GURUMAYI CHIDVILASANANDA
Ashes At My Guru's Feet
Kindle My Heart, Volumes I & II

BY SWAMI MUKTANANDA
From the Finite to the Infinite, Volumes I & II
I Am That
Play of Consciousness
Kundalini: The Secret of Life
Secret of the Siddhas
Siddha Meditation
I Have Become Alive
Does Death Really Exist?
Getting Rid of What You Haven't Got
Where Are You Going?
Light on the Path
Mukteshwari I & II
Satsang With Baba, Volumes I-V
Reflections of the Self
In the Company of a Siddha
Mystery of the Mind
Meditate
I Love You
To Know the Knower
The Self Is Already Attained
A Book for the Mind
I Welcome You All With Love
God Is With You

For more information about Siddha Meditation contact:
Centers Office, SYDA Foundation, P.O. Box 600, South Fallsburg,
New York 12779, (914) 434-2000.

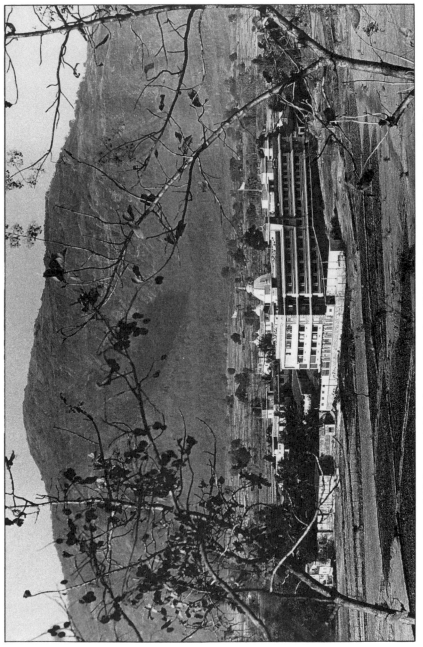

Swami Muktananda's Ashram, Gurudev Siddha Peeth, in Ganeshpuri, India.